An Introduction to Nursing

Theory and Practice

**Mary Henry, Anne Traynor
and Dorothy Phillips**

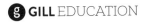

GILL EDUCATION

Gill Education
Hume Avenue
Park West
Dublin 12
www.gilleducation.ie

Gill Education is an imprint of M.H. Gill & Co.

978 07171 6100 3

Design and print origination by O'K Graphic Design, Dublin
Printed by GraphyCems, Spain
Index by Cliff Murphy

For permission to reproduce photographs, the authors and publisher gratefully acknowledge the following:

© Alamy: 91T, 101, 103T, 112, 118, 123CT; © Shutterstock: 9B, 15, 16, 21, 24, 31, 44, 46, 49, 68T, 68B, 69, 72, 73, 74, 76, 79T, 79B, 83C, 90, 91C, 91B, 103B, 104, 119, 123T, 123CB, 123B, 124, 128, 131, 135, 140; © Shutterstock/Neveshkin Nikolay: 1; © World Health Organization 2009. All rights reserved: 83T; Courtesy of An Bord Altranais agus Cnáimhseachais na hÉireann/ Nursing and Midwifery Board of Ireland (NMBI): 3; Courtesy of the Health Service Executive: 9T, 83B, 84, 85, 144, 145, 145, 145, 145, 147.

The authors and publisher have made every effort to trace all copyright holders, but if any has been inadvertently overlooked we would be pleased to make the necessary arrangement at the first opportunity.

The paper used in this book comes from the wood pulp of managed forests. For every tree felled, at least one tree is planted, thereby renewing natural resources.

A CIP catalogue record is available for this book from the British Library.

Carol Kavanagh.

Contents

Preface

This book was written for those teaching and studying the NFQ Level 5 Nursing Studies award. It is written specifically for the module 'Nursing Theory and Practice' and incorporates all of the twelve learning outcomes. The book is relevant to the Irish health setting, however many of the themes are transferable to other care settings.

Nursing Theory and Practice is the core caring module on the Nursing Studies programme and aims to embed in the learner the knowledge and competence to perform a range of basic nursing skills. It also gives learners an introduction to the principles and practice underpinning the Nursing Process and models of nursing.

Many other key areas are included, such as Infection Prevention and Control, Scope of Practice for Nurses and Clinical Skills for Nursing, which provide a good foundation for those thinking of a career in nursing or caring.

Topics such as Models of Nursing, the Nursing Process and Interpersonal Skills introduce the reader to fundamental aspects of nursing which have been reviewed and developed in the profession over a number of decades and will assist in preparing the student for further education in this area.

Overall this book sets out to identify and explore subjects which are vital, relevant and consistent with nursing practice and will help to develop interest and knowledge for anyone teaching or considering a career in the nursing profession.

Development of Nursing as a Profession

LEARNING OBJECTIVES

At the end of this chapter the learner should be able to:

• have an understanding of the development of nursing as a profession in Ireland

Ancient Greeks and ancient Romans

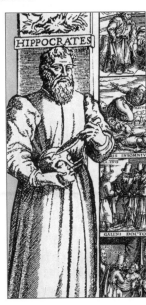

The ancient Greeks are seen by many as being the founders of modern medicine. Hippocrates, a Greek physician, had a very strong influence on the science of medicine. He was the founder of the Hippocratic oath which comprises a set of medical and ethical principles; the Hippocratic oath is still in use today. The ancient Greeks also recognised the link between good hygiene and the promotion of health.

Male physicians in ancient Greece were known as 'iatroi' and had female assistants who had knowledge of the use of herbs in healing. These female healers were seen as assistants to the male physicians who felt the need to dominate their activity to ensure that their primary role as homemakers was undisturbed.

The Romans built upon the knowledge of the Greeks and set about improving sanitation and water systems, as they recognised the link between disease and poor sanitation. Hospitals were built to care for Roman soldiers and nursing care was provided by the wives of noblemen. The Romans also emphasised that people should take care of their own health through exercise and relaxation.

Christianity

With the rise of Christianity in the Roman Empire care was provided by Deacons and Deaconesses within the home environment. The early Christians believed that caring for the sick was an act of love, and care continued to be provided by female members of the sick person's family. The later part of this era saw the development of monasteries, some of which were devoted to caring for the sick and poor.

Ninth to nineteenth centuries

In the Crusades of the ninth century people started to travel over long distances, resulting in a rise in disease transmission. Hospitals were built to care for wounded soldiers and this saw the creation of the Order of St John of God in which men cared for the sick.

During the middle ages the role of women healers was viewed as a threat to their male counterparts which resulted in their playing a subservient role to male physicians (Oakley, 1976).

The reformation resulted in a greater input by religious orders into healthcare. Women working as nurses in the eighteenth and nineteenth centuries had the role of a domestic attendant and care was of a very poor standard. Nursing attracted women who had a basic education and who wished to work (Leddy and Pepper, 1993).

Changes to medicine as a result of scientific progress required further education and training of nurses who worked under the direction of physicians.

Florence Nightingale

Florence Nightingale was a member of the English upper class who believed, after a calling from God, that to care for the sick was her destiny. Florence wished to pursue a career in nursing and despite the disapproval of her parents she spent time working in Germany and later in Paris where she undertook training under the Sisters of Charity order.

She later travelled to the Crimea with other nurses to care for wounded British soldiers and she is credited with improving hygiene standards in the military hospitals.

On her return from the Crimea she set up the Nightingale School of Nursing at St Thomas's hospital, London (Dossey, 2009). Despite her reluctance to allow any input into nurse training from the medical profession, this independent status was not achieved (Bostridge, 2008).

Development of nursing in Ireland

In Ireland the first hospitals were established in the seventeenth century to care for the sick and poor, with the first voluntary hospital opening in Cook Street, Dublin in 1718. Public Infirmaries were developed in rural areas following an act of parliament in 1765.

The Poor Law Act 1838 saw hospitals managed by boards of governors. However standards of hygiene in these buildings were very poor and this resulted in disease transmission.

The Poor Relief Act 1851 saw the establishment of nursing homes and in 1876 a training school for district nurses and midwives was opened. The Sisters of Mercy, Sisters of Charity and Brothers of St John of God also made significant contributions to the improvement of healthcare during this time.

Following the Notification of Births Act (Extension) 1915 nurses were employed to visit children younger than five years in their homes.

The Midwives Act 1918 allowed for the provision of nurse education in Ireland, which in turn led to the establishment of the Central Midwives Board. The General Nursing Council of Ireland was established following the Nurse Registration Act 1919.

An Bord Altranais agus Cnáimhseachais na hÉireann/ Nursing and Midwifery Board of Ireland (NMBI)

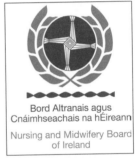

Bord Altranais agus
Cnáimhseachais na hÉireann

Nursing and Midwifery Board
of Ireland

Following the establishment of the Department of Health in 1947 it was recognised that health services would have a vital role in public services in Ireland.

The Nurses Act 1950 allowed for nurses to have a greater say in regulation of their own profession and An Bord Altranais was established, replacing both the General Nursing Council and the Midwives Board (Robins, 2000).

The Report of the Working Party on General Nursing 1980 examined the changing role of the nurse in response to the needs of society and advances in medical technology. The report made recommendations in relation to the restructuring of An Bord Altranais which had changed very little since its formation in 1950.

The Nurses Act 1985 implemented the Working Party Report recommendations, also taking European Union Directives into account at this time. This allowed for the establishment of a new Bord Altranais (Robins, 2000). The main changes to the role and function of the board were as follows:

- Membership of the board was increased from twenty-three to twenty-nine. Seventeen members were from the nursing profession and the remaining twelve appointed by the minister for health.
- A central applications board was established to process all applications for nurse training.
- Registration was updated to include divisions of the register for general nurse, psychiatric nurse, sick children's nurse, mental handicap nurse, midwife, public health nurse and nurse tutor and to allow for recognition of nursing qualifications from member states of the European Union.
- Education and training gave An Bord Altranais the power to approve or withdraw approval to a hospital or healthcare setting to train student nurses and to stipulate minimal educational requirements for entry to nurse training.
- A Fitness to Practise Committee was appointed to sit in judgement on the fitness to practise of nurses in respect of professional misconduct or physical or mental disability.

Functions of An Bord Altranais agus Cnáimhseachais na hÉireann/Nursing and Midwifery Board of Ireland (NMBI)

The NMBI aims to promote high standards of professional education and training and professional conduct among nurses and midwives. In carrying out its regulatory functions, the NMBI aims to protect the public in their dealings with nurses and midwives and protect the integrity of the practice of nursing and midwifery through the promotion of high standards of professional education, training and practice, and professional conduct among nurses and midwives.

The roles and responsibilities of the NMBI in accordance with the Nurses and Midwives Act 2011 are as follows:

- regulation of the nursing and midwifery professions in Ireland
- establishment and maintenance of the register of nurses and midwives and the candidate register
- establishment of procedures and criteria for assessment and registration in the register of nurses and midwives and the candidate register, and the divisions of those registers, including the issue of certificates of registration and renewal of registration
- ensuring the protection of the public in its dealing with nurses and midwives

- promoting and ensuring high standards of professional education, training and practice and professional conduct among nurses and midwives.

In addition to its statutory functions, the NMBI:
- advises the Minister for Health on all matters relating to the functions assigned to the board by the Act
- advises the public on all matters of general interest relating to its functions
- ensures the application of relevant EU Directives in the regulation and control of nursing and midwifery practice
- undertakes additional functions assigned by the Minister for Health in relation to the practice of nursing and midwifery and the persons engaged in such practice
- maintains and fosters relations with relevant international organisations
- provides both library and information services to the professions.

The Commission on Nursing

The *Report of the Commission on Nursing,* which is credited with being the most comprehensive review of nursing and midwifery, was published in 1998. It looked at the evolving role of nurses and midwives working in the health services taking into account issues such as professional development, the nurse's role in the management of services, promotional opportunities, training and educational requirements and the role and function of An Bord Altranais.

Four main recommendations were made by the Commission:
- the establishment of the Nursing Education Forum (for pre-registration education)
- the establishment of the National Council (for post-registration education)
- the establishment of Nursing and Midwifery Planning and Development Units (NMPDU) in each health board area
- the introduction of legislation amending the 1985 Nurses Act (The Nurses and Midwives Act 2011)

The first three recommendations were introduced within two years of the publication of the report, with the fourth taking until 2011.

The report provided a plan for the development of the professions into the future. Two major recommendations were the introduction of a pre-registration degree programme and the development of structured clinical career pathways for nurses and midwives (O'Shea, 2013).

Nursing and midwifery education

The education programmes for nurses and midwives were totally changed following recommendations of the *Report of the Commission on Nursing* 1998.

Prior to this, general, psychiatric and intellectual disability nurse training was a three-year apprenticeship model which was hospital-based, consisting of classroom instruction and hands-on practical training under the direction of nursing tutors in the training hospital. Assessment was continuous with a final written examination conducted by the NMBI.

Following a review by the NMBI this model of training was changed to a diploma-based programme in general, psychiatric and intellectual disability nursing which was introduced on a pilot basis in Galway in 1994 and rolled out to the rest of the country over the following four years.

Following on recommendations of the *Report of the Commission on Nursing* the diploma programme was changed to the current four-year degree programme commencing in 2002 with applications through the CAO, in line with all other degree courses.

In 2006 direct entry to the midwifery four-year degree and the four-and-a-half-year integrated children's and general nursing degree programmes commenced. Entry to both of these courses had previously been post-registration only (O'Shea, 2013).

Post-registration education

Currently there are five post-registration programmes leading to additional registration with the NMBI: children's nursing, midwifery, nurse tutor, public health nursing and nurse prescriber.

Nurses and Midwives Act 2011

The Nurses and Midwives Act 2011 was signed into legislation on 21 December 2011. The NMBI is currently working on all projects necessary to implement the new Act in consultation with specific stakeholders.

The Act aims to enhance the protection of the public in dealings with nurses and midwives, while ensuring the integrity of these professional groups.

The Act will allow for fitness-to-practise inquiries to be held in public in the majority of cases to allow for a more transparent system of dealing with complaints.

A review of the Code of Professional Conduct is also being undertaken to support professional guidance.

The Act recognises midwifery as a separate and distinct profession to that of nursing and to allow for this the name of the board has changed to An Bord Altranais agus Cnáimhseachais na hÉireann, or Nursing and Midwifery Board of Ireland (NMBI).

> **ACTIVITY**
>
> Research the following:
> * the clinical career pathways for nurses and midwives post pre-registration training (to CNS/CMS/ANP/AMP)
> * the management career pathways for nurses and midwives (to CNM/CMM)

Revision

1. Draw a mind map to trace the development of the nursing profession from the ancient Greeks and Romans to where nursing is today.
2. What influences did the religious orders and Florence Nightingale have on the development of nursing?
3. What were the main recommendations made by the *Report of the Commission on Nursing*?
4. What are the functions of the NMBI?

References

NMBI, 'Bord functions' available at www.nursingboard.ie/en/ab-board_functions.aspx (2013) (accessed 29/08/2013).

Bostridge, B., *Florence Nightingale: The Woman and her Legend*, London: Viking 2008.

Dossey, B., *Florence Nightingale: Mystic, Visionary, Healer*, Philadelphia: F. A. Davis Company 2009.

Government of Ireland, *Nurses Act 1985*, Dublin: Stationery Office 1985.

Government of Ireland, *Nurses and Midwives Act 2011*, Dublin: Stationary Office 2011.

Government of Ireland, *Report of the Commission on Nursing: A Blueprint for the Future*, Dublin: Stationery Office 1998.

Government of Ireland, *The Nurses Registration Act 1919*, Dublin: Stationery Office 1919.

Leddy, S. and Pepper, J., *Conceptual Basis of Professional Nursing*, 3rd ed., Philadelphia: Lippincott 1993.

Oakley, A., *A Social History of Medicine*, London: Longman 1976.

O'Shea, Y., *The Professional Development of Nursing and Midwifery in Ireland: Key Challenges for the Twenty-First Century*, Dublin: Orpen Press 2013.

Robins, J., *Nursing and Midwifery in Ireland in the Twentieth Century*, Dublin: An Bord Altranais 2000.

Health Services in Ireland

At the end of this chapter the learner should be able to:

- **have an understanding of the healthcare structures and functions in Ireland**
- **explain primary, acute and tertiary care**
- **understand the effects of European Union Directives on nursing**

Health services evolution

It was not until the late 1940s that health was viewed as a priority for Irish governments. The Department of Health was established in 1947. Prior to this health in Ireland was dealt with by the Department of Local Government and Public Health with health services being administered through local authorities. The Health Act 1970 saw control of health services removed from local authorities and reorganised into eight regional Health Boards reporting to the Department of Health. It also gave provision for the establishment of the Regional Hospitals and Comhairle na nOspidéal (the Hospital Council) creating a regional structure for healthcare (Barrington, 1987).

The publication of the health strategy *Shaping a Healthier Future: A Strategy for Effective Healthcare in the 1990s* paved the way for further reform of the health service. The strategy was based on three principles: equity, quality and accountability, and was developed following a number of reports commissioned by the Department of Health.

In 2001 the re-named Department of Health and Children published a new strategy, *Quality and Fairness: A Health System for You*. This document added a fourth principle – people centredness – to the three principles of equity, quality and accountability of the earlier strategy *Shaping a Healthier Future*.

A number of further studies were commissioned by the government and following evaluation of these the Health Service Reform Programme was introduced in 2003.

The Health Act of 2004 saw the establishment of the Health Service Executive (HSE) which came into operation in January 2005 (O'Shea, 2013).

The Health Service Executive

The Health Service Executive (HSE) plans and delivers publically funded health and social services for people in the Republic of Ireland.

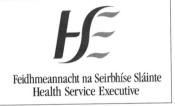

Feidhmeannacht na Seirbhíse Sláinte
Health Service Executive

The Integrated Services Directorate of the HSE manages all hospital and community public health services in Ireland and has overall responsibility for the delivery of all health and personal social services in Ireland including hospital, primary, community and continuing care services.

Health services provided by the HSE are managed currently within four regions: HSE Dublin North East, HSE Dublin Mid-Leinster, HSE West and HSE South.

Each of the four regions is subdivided into a number of HSE areas, with each area having an area manager who oversees the provision of health and social services in hospitals and communities.

Services provided within a HSE area include acute hospital services, primary care services, mental health services, child care services, disability services, social inclusion services, elderly/nursing home services, dental services and a range of allowances including Supplementary Welfare Allowance, Domiciliary Care Allowance, Blind Welfare Allowance, Mobility Allowance etc.

Primary care

Primary care services are all of the health or social care services that are delivered in the community and outside of the hospital setting. Primary care includes GPs, public health nurses and a range of other services provided through a local health office.

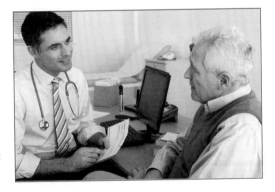

Professionals working in primary care include:

- GP and practice nurses
- community paediatric services
- community nursing service – public health nurses, community registered nurses
- occupational therapists
- physiotherapists
- home help/support staff

The primary care team members also link with other community-based disciplines such as

- mental health services
- counsellors and psychologists
- social workers
- podiatrists
- dental services
- ophthalmic services
- dieticians
- speech and language therapists

Acute hospitals

Acute hospital services diagnose, treat and care for seriously ill or injured patients, and are provided in HSE hospitals, public voluntary hospitals and private hospitals. Some hospitals have specialist care, for example maternity or psychiatric hospitals, while others are of a general nature.

The large general and regional hospitals provide a broad range of services, while smaller local hospitals may not have the resources to cater for all illnesses and treatments and may have to transfer patients to regional or specialist hospitals.

ACTIVITY

Make a list of the professional staffing groups who work at your local hospital and research their specific roles and responsibilities.

Now make a list of all other staff (non-professional) who work at the hospital and research their specific roles.

In May 2013 Minister for Health James Reilly announced a reorganisation of public hospitals into what have been described as more efficient and accountable hospital groups that will deliver improved patient outcomes.

The six new hospital groups which will comprise between six and eleven hospitals, to include one major teaching hospital, will be as follows:

- Dublin North East
- Dublin Midlands
- Dublin East

- South/South West
- West/North West
- Midwest

Tertiary care

Tertiary care is specialised consultative health care, usually for inpatients that have been referred from a primary or secondary health facility/source. Tertiary care is delivered in a facility that has personnel and resources for advanced medical investigation and treatment. Examples of tertiary care services are cardiac surgery, neurosurgery, cancer management, plastic surgery, treatment of severe burns, transplantation surgery and many other complex surgical and medical interventions.

> **ACTIVITY**
>
> Research two tertiary referral centres in Ireland.
> Are either/both in your health region?
> What type of tertiary care is provided?
> What professional staffing groups work in these centres?

European Union Directives and nursing in Ireland

European Union Directives relating to general nurses were first introduced in 1977 (Directives 77/452/EEC and 77/453/EEC) and relating to midwifery in 1980 (Directives 80/154/EEC and 80/155/EEC) and have been amended over time to allow for changes. They harmonised general nursing education programmes throughout the European Union by setting out the minimum duration and content for such programmes.

European Union member states were mandated to comply with these minimum requirements, and provisions were set out whereby general nurses or midwives who were educated and trained in one member state could gain registration in another member state.

Nurses in other divisions of the Register such as psychiatric nurses, children's nurses, intellectual disability nurses, public health nurses and nurse tutors can apply to have their application to register in another member state assessed, as education was not harmonised in these divisions.

Directive 2005/36/EC made no changes to the duration and content of nursing and midwifery programmes. Under this directive the NMBI must recognise the qualifications of nurses and midwives educated and trained in member states and in certain circumstances recognise individuals educated and trained in non-European countries, but who have been recognised in another member state.

Revision

1. Discuss the difference between primary, acute and tertiary care.
2. What types of services are provided by primary care?
3. What types of professionals work in the primary care setting?
4. Research what type of care each professional you have listed provides.
5. What are the effects of European Directives on nursing?
6. What changes were proposed in 2013 for the reorganisation of public hospitals?

References

Barrington, R., *Health, Medicine and Politics in Ireland 1900–1970*, Dublin: Institute of Public Administration 1987.

Department of Health, *Quality and Fairness: A Health System for You*, Dublin: Department of Health 2001.

Department of Health, *Shaping a Healthier Future: A Strategy for Effective Healthcare in the 1990s,* Dublin: Department of Health and Children 1994.

European Communities (Recognition of General Nursing Qualifications) Regulations, 1980 (S.I. No. 237 of 1980).

European Communities (Recognition of Midwifery Nursing Qualifications) Regulations, 1983 (S.I. No. 20 of 1983).

European Communities (Recognition of Professional Qualifications of Nurses and Midwives) Regulations, 2008 (S.I. No. 164 of 2008).

Government of Ireland, *Health Act 1970,* Dublin: Stationary Office 1970.

Government of Ireland, *Health Act 2004,* Dublin: Stationary Office 2004.

O'Shea, Y., *The Professional Development of Nursing and Midwifery in Ireland: Key Challenges for the Twenty-First Century*, Dublin: Orpen Press 2013.

3

The Code of Professional Conduct and Scope of Practice

LEARNING OBJECTIVES

At the end of this chapter the learner should be able to:

- outline the Code of Professional Conduct for each Nurse and Midwife in Ireland
- outline the Scope of Nursing and Midwifery Practice Framework in Ireland

Code of Professional Conduct for each Nurse and Midwife (April 2000)

The purpose of the code of conduct is to provide guidance to nurses and midwives in professional decision-making and in carrying out their responsibilities while promoting high standards of professional conduct.

Nurses and midwives are expected to exhibit high standards of professional behaviour at all times with each nurse and midwife being accountable for their own practice.

The *Code of Professional Conduct* and *Scope of Practice* are currently under review by the NMBI with a view to publishing a new code of professional conduct and ethics for registered nurses and midwives in the near future.

The following are the main elements of the current code of conduct.

Provide the highest standard of care to patients

The nursing profession aims to provide the highest standard of care possible to patients. Unsafe standards of care should be reported to the appropriate persons or authorities by the nurse or midwife.

Confidentiality

Information regarding a patient's history, health status and treatment is privileged and confidential. The nurse or midwife must use their professional judgement and responsibility in sharing this information with colleagues and confidentiality of patients' records must be safeguarded.

Where a nurse or midwife is called to give evidence in court legal advice should be sought to ensure compliance with confidentiality.

Informed judgement and consent

The nurse or midwife should ensure that patients understand the nature and purpose of any treatment before consent is sought. Withholding information in certain circumstances should be undertaken with due care.

Sexual advances

Any form of sexual advance to a patient where a professional relationship exists is considered misconduct.

Competence

The nurse or midwife must practise within their own scope of practice and must take measures to develop and maintain the necessary competence for professional practice. Any limitations in competence must be acknowledged by the nurse or midwife and he or she must refuse to undertake delegated or assigned tasks for which he or she is not competent.

Conscientious objections

Conscientious objections relevant to professional practice should be made known to the appropriate persons at the earliest opportunity.

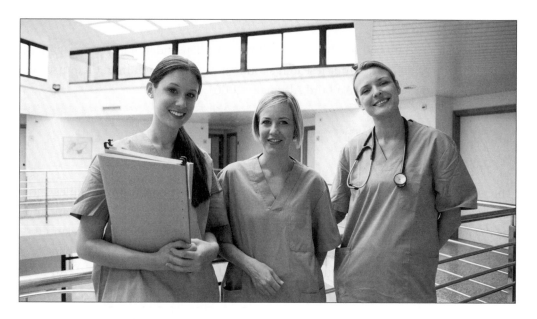

Junior colleagues and students

Tasks should only be assigned to junior colleagues and students that are within their scope of practice. The nurse or midwife has a responsibility to share acquired knowledge and skill with junior colleagues and students. The nurse or midwife has overall responsibility for care provided by students under their supervision.

Preservation of human life

Every effort to preserve human life should be made and in situations where death is imminent care should be taken to ensure the patient's dignity.

Public statements

It should always be clearly stated whether the nurse or midwife is speaking in a personal or professional capacity. The promotion of commercial products should be avoided in order that professional judgement in not compromised.

Gifts or favours

Gifts or favours that may compromise professional practice should be declined.

Personal health and welfare

Attention should be given to personal health in order not to compromise practice, to include the abuse of alcohol or drugs.

Nursing research

Ethical policies and procedure should be adhered to when undertaking or engaging in research. Permission to carry out research should always be sought from the nurse's or midwife's appropriate body (An Bord Altranais, 2000).

Scope of Nursing and Midwifery Practice Framework

'The term Scope of Practice refers to the range of roles, functions, responsibilities and activities, which a registered nurse, or registered midwife is educated, competent, and has the authority to perform. Scope of practice for nurses and midwives in Ireland is determined by legislation, EU directives, international developments, social policy, national and local guidelines, education and individual levels of competence' (An Bord Altranais, 2000).

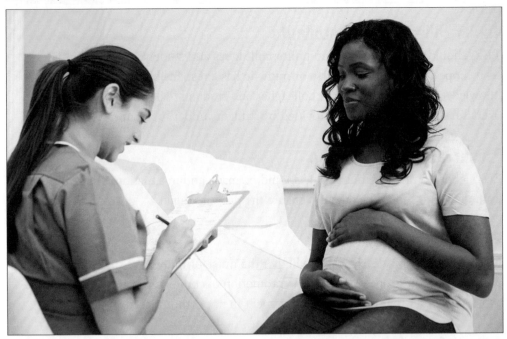

Key considerations that the nurse or midwife should consider in determining their scope of practice include:

Competence

- Is the nurse or midwife competent to carry out their particular role or function?
- Measures should be taken to maintain competence for professional practice.

Accountability and autonomy

Accountability

- The nurse or midwife is answerable for decisions made in the course of professional practice, to include both actions and omissions.

- Nurses and midwives are accountable both professionally and legally.

Autonomy

- Accountability can only be achieved when the nurse or midwife has the autonomy to practice.

- Nurses and midwives can make professional decisions and act on them within their scope of practice.

Continuous professional development

- Nurses and midwives are required to undertake continuous professional development in order to maintain professional standards.

- The responsibility to develop professionally lies with the individual nurse or midwife.

Support for professional nursing and midwifery practice

- Nursing and midwifery managers need to ensure that systems are in place to support professional practice through national and local guidelines, policies and protocols.

Delegation

- Delegation should only occur when the nurse or midwife is confident that the person assigned to carry out the task has the competence and skills necessary and that delegation serves the best interests of the patient.

Emergency situations

- The scope of practice should not deter the nurse or midwife from taking appropriate action in the case of an emergency, where such action is in the patient's best interest.

(An Bord Altranais, 2000)

Both the *Code of Professional Conduct* and the *Scope of Practice* can be viewed and downloaded from www.nursingboard.ie and as both documents are currently under review any changes made will be published on the site.

ACTIVITY

Confidentiality and security

Fairdale is an 80-bed residential unit for the elderly. All patient records are held in paper format and are stored in folders in a locked trolley in the clinical nurse manager's office.

One evening Mrs Brown is found crying by the nurse caring for her. She says that her folder with all of her medical information was handed to her by another concerned resident who had found it lying on a coffee table in the foyer of the unit.

She says she has read the file and is upset as she read that her hospital appointment next week for weight loss and tiredness is to investigate the possibility of leukaemia.

Mrs Brown is angry as she had not received any results of recent blood tests and had asked that same morning and was told that no results were back yet. She becomes very distressed as she wants to know why she 'has not been told the truth'.

1. What are the confidentiality and security issues in this case?
2. Read over the code of conduct again; are there any areas of concern relating to this case study?
3. How can staff respond to Mrs Brown's immediate distress?
4. What actions need to be taken? (Consider both immediate actions and long-term actions.)

Revision

1. List and write short notes on the guidelines within the code of conduct.
2. In the scope of practice what do the following terms mean?
   i) competence
   ii) autonomy
   iii) accountability
3. How does having a code of conduct and scope of practice enhance the nursing profession and in particular the professional relationship with patients?

References

An Bord Altranais, *The Code of Professional Conduct for each Nurse and Midwife*, Dublin: Stationery Office 2000.

An Bord Altranais, *Review of Scope of Practice for Nursing and Midwifery – Final Report*, Dublin: Stationery Office 2000.

4

The Nursing Process

The Nursing Process

The Nursing Process is a dynamic, systematic, goal-orientated framework for problem-solving that helps the nurse to plan care for the patient while promoting critical thinking. It is cost efficient and is part of the standard of care in nursing. The Nursing Process enhances the quality of decisions made and promotes professionalism in nursing, while increasing patient participation, enhancing communication and improving efficiency of care.

What is critical thinking?

Critical thinking is when the nurse thinks about their own thoughts and what they say, write and do, in addition to what others say, write and do. While thinking about all of this they are questioning the appropriateness of their actions, applying nursing standards and seeing how things measure up. Alternatively the nurse may be thinking about alternative ways of handling a situation (Brookfield, 1991).

Purposes of the Nursing Process

The Nursing Process has many purposes. Its primary aim is to provide a systematic method for nursing practice. In addition it unifies, standardises and directs nursing practice (Christensen, 1995). It is a thought and procedure process.

The Nursing Process

- enhances communication

- is an educational tool
- increases patient participation in care
- promotes continuity of care
- facilitates documentation
- improves efficiency
- promotes critical thinking
- gives direction to nursing practice

Stages of the Nursing Process

In 1967 Yura and Walsh established a number of stages in the Nursing Process and advocated a more systematic and analytical approach to patient care (Aggleton, 1992).

There are currently five stages of the Nursing Process and it is important to know the purpose of each stage.

The acronym ADPIE may help you to remember the stages in order:

1. Assessment
2. Diagnosis
3. Planning
4. Implementation
5. Evaluation

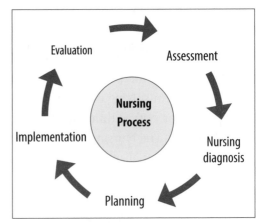

Assessment

During this stage the nurse has their initial contact with the patient and establishes a database of the patient's healthcare needs and their ability to manage their needs. During this stage the nurse gathers information about the patient in a systematic, organised way.

The assessment stage is systematic and continuous and is a vital part of the Nursing Process as all other stages rely on valid and complete data collected and documented at this point.

During the assessment the nurse

- collects data
- organises data
- validates data
- documents data

Subjective and objective data

Data collected is defined as either subjective or objective and it is important to be able to distinguish between the two.

Subjective data

This may be described as symptoms or other information that the patient gives you, for example a description of their pain.

Objective data

This is data that can be measured or tested against an accepted standard. Objective data can be seen, heard, felt or smelt. It is obtained through observation or physical assessment (for example the patient's pulse rate or blood pressure measurement).

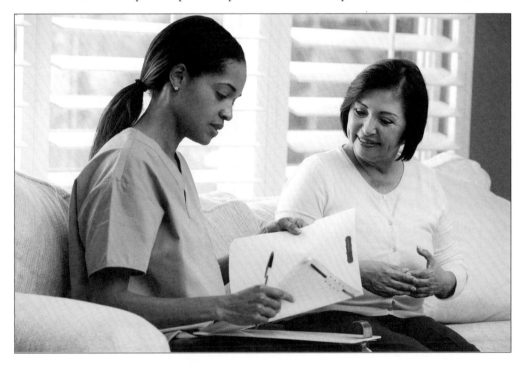

Methods of data collection

Data can be collected through the following methods:

Observation

The nurse uses the five senses to gather data.

Interviewing

An interview is a structured form of communication. Prior to the interview the nurse should explain the purpose of the interview and provide privacy and comfort while ensuring confidentiality. Both open and closed questions are used while always making sure that the patient is comfortable with the process.

Physical examination

A head-to-toe approach is often used to avoid data omission and in addition a review of body systems may be carried out by the nurse.

The following are some of the elements noted, measured and recorded:

- observation of general health status
- vital signs (temperature, pulse, respiration and blood pressure)
- weight
- urinalysis
- skin, hair and nails
- dress
- hygiene
- nutritional status
- mobility evaluation
- posture
- mood
- hearing and sight (do there appear to be any issues?)
- bowel elimination
- urine elimination
- language and memory
- circulation
- oedema
- social data
- lifestyle
- spiritual data

It is important to remember to see the person as a whole and not just a review of body systems or a head-to-toe checklist as above. These are merely designed to avoid omissions during the assessment phase and not in any way to dehumanise the patient.

The nurse should also note any signs of distress, wincing or breathing difficulties etc.

A complete health history is reviewed and recorded taking into account information such as biographical data, history of present illness, previous medical history, family history, known allergies, current and past medication and the patient's perception of their current health status.

Data gathering

Data can be obtained from primary and secondary sources.

Primary sources

This is data gathered or obtained directly from the patient themselves. In the majority of incidences data gathered from the patient is considered to be the most reliable source. However in cases where this may not be possible due to age, mental status or the seriousness of the illness a secondary source may be used.

Secondary sources

Secondary sources may be family members, previous medical, laboratory and nursing records and information obtained from other health professionals.

Data validation

Information gathered must be accurate, factual and complete as the nurse will base their diagnosis and intervention on this data.

Validation involves double checking the information collected to ensure that it is accurate and factual. Any discrepancies noted should be reviewed by the nurse before proceeding to the next step in the process.

Documenting data

To complete the assessment stage the nurse should document the patient's data in the nursing notes. Accurate documentation is essential as this forms part of the patient's healthcare record.

Data is always recorded in a factual manner, for example 'Lunch: 150 mls soup, 1 slice brown bread, 100 mls tea' **rather than** 'not hungry so very light lunch taken'.

Assessment is not a step that is undertaken once and not repeated. It is required at any time when there is a change in the patient's status, and is required continually in any rapidly changing situation. Responsibility for assessment is not just the duty of the admitting nurse but is shared across the entire nursing team caring for the patient.

However the first assessment will be used and updated by many nurses during the patient's stay, so accurate, concise, clear and up-to-date data is required.

ACTIVITY

Using role play in a group of four, take a nursing history using the case study below. One member of the group should act as the nurse, another as the patient and the remaining two members observe, taking notes and giving constructive feedback after the activity is completed.

Case study

Mary Smith

Mary is a 76-year-old lady admitted to your hospital following an unexplained fall. She has had X-rays which confirm a fractured hip and she will be listed for surgery tomorrow morning. She has Type 2 diabetes and appears agitated and is pulling on her IV cannula. She lives alone and has one son.

Diagnosis

The nursing diagnosis is the nurse's clinical judgement about the patient's response to actual or potential health problems or needs; it is a vital element of the process and forms the basis for the nurse's care plan. A clear diagnosis enhances communication between team members. It is important to remember that nurses do not make medical diagnoses, for example 'chest infection', but do however use an international standardised language for making clinical judgements, for example dyspnoea (shortness of breath), activity intolerance, cyanosis etc.

Actual and potential health problems are identified and priorities are established through the following stages:

- Analysis of data: data collected during the assessment stage is categorised and investigated to highlight significant signs and symptoms.

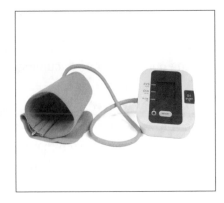

- Interpretation of data: all the various pieces of the puzzle are placed together so that signs, potential causes and correct problem-identification become clear.

- Formulation of the problem statement: the nurse draws conclusions based on signs, pointers and possible causes.

Actual and potential health problems

Actual problems	Potential problems
A problem that is present at the time of the nursing assessment, for example acute pain or breathlessness.	Evidence about the health problem is incomplete or unclear or the problem is considered only a possibility, for example risk of constipation due to inactivity or insufficient fluid intake.

As the nursing problem statement forms the basis for the planning, implementation and evaluation stages, care should be taken to ensure concise, accurate information is documented (Basford, 1999).

Planning

During this stage a care plan is written in order to plan how to achieve outcomes or solve problems identified in the assessment and diagnosis stages.

It is important that priorities are established with immediate attention given to any life-threatening issues, then non-life threatening issues and lastly potential problems that may arise. Remember that reassessment of needs is required as the patient's health status changes.

The nursing care plan must clearly specify who will effect the desired outcome, the actions required and a time-frame. Outcomes are often describes as goals. The individualised care plan is stored in the nursing records.

A commonly used framework to help the nurses identify problems is Maslow's Hierarchy of Needs, with physiological needs requiring first priority. This incorporates life-threatening issues that pose a threat to physiological needs.

Maslow's Hierarchy of Needs

Once all physiological needs are identified and goals established, the nurse moves on to the next stage, identifying needs for safety and security, and so on up to the final stage of self-actualisation.

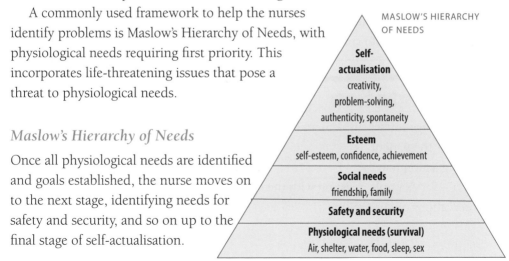

MASLOW'S HIERARCHY OF NEEDS

Self-actualisation
creativity, problem-solving, authenticity, spontaneity

Esteem
self-esteem, confidence, achievement

Social needs
friendship, family

Safety and security

Physiological needs (survival)
Air, shelter, water, food, sleep, sex

Establishing goals

Goals give direction to nursing actions and a focus for the evaluation stage. Goals can be short-term or long-term depending on the problem identified. They are written in a clear, non-ambiguous manner in the care plan and communicated to the rest of the team.

Goals need to be SMART

- **S**pecific (clear and detailed for everyone to understand)
- **M**easurable (be specific: what changes will you see?)
- **A**chievable (is the goal possible given the patient's health status or healthcare resources?)
- **R**elevant (is it realistic?)
- **T**ime-limited (deadlines motivate, but need to be realistic)

(College of Nurses of Ontario, 2012)

The written care plan should identify and communicate all action to be delivered to meet the patient's care needs.

ACTIVITY

Mrs Johnson fell while walking to the bathroom in your ward at 3 a.m. You did not witness the fall but were alerted by another patient. She appears to have hit her head and there is a large amount of blood coming from a wound to the side of her left ear. She is crying and complaining of pain in her left arm which she tells you she cannot move. The left arm appears to be at an odd angle to her body.

What are your priorities in caring for Mrs Johnson?

Give reasons for your choices.

Implementation

During this stage nurses implement the individualised care plan that has been prepared for the patient.

Nursing action may be

- direct – for example assisting with the activities of daily living, teaching, observations or counselling

- indirect – performed away from the patient but on their behalf, for example advocacy or supervision

Evaluation

This is the final stage in the Nursing Process and can only take place when all other stages have been implemented. During this stage the nurse reviews the nursing interventions or actions and decides if they have met the desired outcomes identified in the care plan.

Questions the nurse needs to consider include:

- Have goals been met?
- If not, why not?
- Does the plan need to be altered or amended?
- Did the patient's health status change?
- Were the goals realistic and achievable?

Evaluation is an ongoing process designed to improve patient care by systematically reviewing the results of nursing care against each goal set in the care plan. It involves both practical knowledge and evidence-based research in order to identify appropriate outcomes. Through evaluation both the nurse and patient can gain an understanding of what goals have or have not been achieved.

Critical thinking plays an important role here, to differentiate between appropriate outcomes and actual outcomes.

Revision

1. What are the five stages of the Nursing Process?
2. Describe the nurse's action at each stage.
3. How does each stage relate and contribute to patient care?
4. What does critical thinking involve?
5. What is the difference between objective and subjective data?
6. What are SMART goals?
7. State the difference between actual and potential health problems.
8. Look at Maslow's Hierarchy of Needs and list possible nursing care priorities at each stage.

References

Aggleton, P. and Chalmers, H., *Nursing Models and the Nursing Process*, 2nd ed., London: Macmillan 1992.

Basford, L. *et al.*, *Theory and Practice of Nursing*, Cheltenham: Stanley Thornes 1999.

Brookfield, S. D., *Developing Critical Thinkers*, San Francisco: Jossey Bass 1991.

Christensen, P. and Kenney, J., *Nursing Process: Application of Conceptual Models*, 4th ed., New York: Mosby Year Books 1995.

College of Nurses of Ontario, 'Developing SMART learning goals' available at www. cno.org/Global/docs/qa/DevelopingSMARTGoals.pdf (2012).

5

Models of Nursing

At the end of this chapter the learner should be able to:

- **explain what is meant by a theory and model of nursing**
- **explain the purpose of the nursing models**
- **outline the main features of at least two models of nursing**
- **identify how the application of models to practice influences the activity of the nurse and the experience for the patient or client**
- **name the twelve activities of living**
- **identify factors which influence the activities of living**
- **use questions to assess individuals' needs using the activities of living**

Models of nursing

Nursing models have been developed by nurse theorists since the 1960s. It is claimed that nursing models and theories helped nursing to evolve from a task-oriented activity to a logical and systematic approach to care, and that they guide practice (Pearson *et al.*, 1996). Nursing theory exists to improve practice as it expresses the values and beliefs of nursing, creating a structure in which to organise knowledge and illuminate nursing practice (Parker and Smith, 2010). Models of nursing outline a framework for nursing care that is systematically constructed and of scientific origin (Fawcett, 1995).

There has been much criticism of models for over-use of jargon (Kenny, 1993; Hodgson, 1992). Miller (1984) argued that models were idealistic and lacked relevance to the reality of nursing practice, implying that nurses were less likely to use them so that models increased the gap between theory and practice. However Murphy (2010) argues that some of this criticism arose from a lack of understanding of the aim and purpose of nursing models and their implementation, rather than from the concepts and ideas within them, and therefore nursing models may contain basic concepts, values and beliefs about nursing that are important in modern-day nursing.

This chapter outlines what a theory and a model of nursing is and explains the idea of concepts which form theories and models. It will also outline the basic components of three nursing models, focusing in detail on Roper, Logan and Tierney's Activities of Living nursing model.

What is a theory?

According to Chinn and Kramer (2004:268) a theory 'is a creative and rigorous structuring of ideas that projects a tentative, purposeful and systematic view of phenomena'. A theory therefore is a rational or clear proposal which summarises and explains a group of ideas or a philosophy which has been derived from research or observation; it outlines concepts or ideas and highlights similarities between them. Therefore a theory supports the development of knowledge, helps professionals set goals and reach evidence-based conclusions based on observation, explains and predicts outcomes and supports decision-making.

Concepts behind nursing theory

Concepts are fundamentally images or words that portray ideas and describe objects and are basic components of theory. A metaparadigm is a concept that is general; one that serves to define an entire world of thought. 'Meta', in Greek, means 'that which is behind', and refers to that which underpins something else.

Many people have set out to explain 'what nursing is', among them Florence Nightingale, as the founder of modern nursing, who is credited for sowing the seeds of theoretical development in nursing, as well as separating nursing from medicine. Nightingale introduced concepts such as the need to focus on the wellbeing of the individual, the importance of the interaction with the environment and the process by which positive health changes occur (Parker and Smith, 2010).

Facwett (1984), a well-respected nurse theorist, described a metaparadigm of four central elements which sets out to underpin the concepts of nursing. This metaparadigm consists of four concepts; person, environment, health and nursing and she claimed that nursing is the study of the interrelationship between these concepts, which are outlined on the next page.

Person receiving the care

Fawcett (1984) refers to the sick individual not as a 'patient' but as a 'subject', who should be viewed as a whole, unique person taking into account culture, family and role within society.

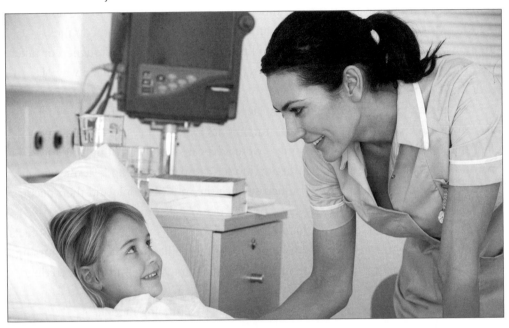

State of health at the time of interaction with the patient

It is difficult to define health for a healthy individual. Health is very general and can vary according to the day and condition of the patient. Health is not a concrete concept, but exists in the context of the health problems of the individual. A person suffering with chronic illness may consider a healthy day as one where they do not have great pain or suffering.

Environment in which the individual exists

This concept is vital as it is about all the elements that will promote recovery of the patient. It includes the individual's mental state, attitudes, experience, home life, physical pain, chances of relapse, state of work and play and a host of other variables which define the context of recovery.

Appropriate nursing actions

This refers to any treatment provided by the nurse to the patient. It includes not just physical care but also ethics, compassion, emotional care and promotion of the general wellbeing of the individual.

What is a model of nursing?

In very simple terms, a model can be thought of as a way of representing reality. Models can be physical, such as a skeleton which represents the human body or a model car which represents a particular brand of car. Models allows people to familiarise themselves with an object, understand it, and take it apart to see how it works (Murphy *et al.*, 2010). Models can also represent abstract and complex situations, such as states of health or disability. While they cannot be touched or taken apart they can be drawn or illustrated and represent a real and systematic way of working or completing a task.

The Nursing Process, as developed by Henderson, is considered to be a vehicle for using models of nursing in practical nursing. Its logical processes – assessing, planning, implementing and evaluating – were advocated as a way of putting into operation the concepts used in the nursing models (Roper, Logan and Tierney, 2005).

Nursing models, influenced by human science theories of people and their needs, suggest ways of improving nursing care and practice (Aggleton and Chalmers, 1992). Models enable us to explore how the nature of nursing is defined. Models are not facts – they evolve and inform thinking and work within the different processes of nursing.

Nursing models are generally identified using the name of the individual credited with developing them.

At a basic level, there are three key components to a nursing model:

* a set of beliefs and values

* a statement of the goal the nurse is trying to achieve

* the knowledge and skills the nurse needs to practise (Pearson et al., 1996)

According to O'Connor (2002), a nursing model should give direction to nurses working in a particular area, as it should help them understand the logic behind their actions. It should also help in decision-making and allow for more co-operation within the team of nurses as a whole. This in turn should lead to continuity and consistency of the nursing care received by patients (Pearson *et al.*, 1996). Different models are used in different areas. There are many nursing models in use, including Neuman's Systems Model and Watson's Theory of Caring. The following nursing models are discussed in this book:

* Roy's Adaptation Model

* Orem's Self-Care Deficit Model

* Roper, Logan and Tierney's Activity of Living

The difference between models and theories

Theories	Models
Built from a set of concepts and ideas that are related.	Built from a set of concepts and ideas that are related; when used in conjunction with a tool such as the Nursing Process they can be applied in practical care situations.
There are not as many theories of nursing as there are models.	Many models of varying quality and focus have been developed.
Theories are considered to be more powerful as they can explain behaviour or issues central to nursing such as the metaparadigm mentioned on page 30. Theories can be considered to be the tried and tested nursing models.	Models contain the seeds of ideas which may be developed and amalgamated with other concepts to eventually form a theory.
Theories are considered to be specific, more defined and factual and have obvious links between ideas.	Models are abstract and can be nonrepresentational or speculative.

Source: Adapted from Aggleton and Chalmers (1992).

The Roy Adaptation Model

The Roy Adaptation Model provides a framework for nursing practice with individuals and groups as well as designing nursing care systems. It was introduced in 1970 by Sister Callista Roy, a nurse theorist, writer, lecturer, researcher and teacher. It continues to be used in nursing today (Parker and Smith, 2010).

The model suggests

The person is in constant interaction with a changing environment and needs mechanisms which they are born with and which they develop to adapt and cope with the changing environment. Health and illness are part of the person's life. The person must adapt to be able to respond positively to environmental changes.

- The person is a biological, psychological and social being who is made up of systems.
- A person's circumstances determine the level the person can adapt to change; health is gained by adapting positively to the environment.
- Each individual has four modes of adaptation: physiologic needs, self-concept, role function and inter-dependence.

- Treating people as individuals in a holistic manner is extremely important for nursing.
- Interaction and interpersonal relations are fundamental to nursing.
- Individuals aim to exist within society with the ultimate goal of achieving integrity and dignity.

There are different levels of assessment of behaviour. The first involves gathering data about the behaviour of the person or group as an adaptive system and the second is the assessment of stimuli that influence the behaviour. A nursing diagnosis is then made. Following this, in collaboration with the individual or group, the adaptation level is classified as integrated, compensatory or compromised. Goals are set establishing clear statements of behavioural outcomes. Intervention focuses on helping the individual reach the established goals, and evaluation involves judging the effectiveness of the nursing intervention (Parker and Smith, 2010).

Orem's Self-Care Deficit Model

Dorothea E. Orem (1914–2007) developed the Self-Care Deficit nursing model. It comprises three minor interrelated theories; theory of self-care, theory of self-care deficit and theory of nursing systems. Orem considered there were two types of humans; those that need care and those that produce it; put simply, the patient and the nurse (Parker and Smith, 2010).

The model suggests

Individuals should be encouraged to be independent and responsible for their own care and that of other family members who need care; there is a collective responsibility to maintain health.

- All people are unique individuals.
- Nursing is an interaction between two or more persons.
- Promoting an accepted level of independence and promoting self-care are important parts of primary care and prevention of ill health.
- A person's own perspective and knowledge of their health is important and should be part of the assessment.
- A person's knowledge of potential health problems is necessary for promoting independence and self-care behaviours.
- Self-care and dependent care are behaviours learned within society and can vary according to cultural habits and practice.

- Using a tool such as the Nursing Process and the components of this model an individual's problems and potential problems are identified and a plan is made with a focus on goals which promote self-care rather than dependency on the nursing system.

Roper, Logan and Tierney: Activities of Living Nursing Model

TABLE 1

Activities of living
1.	Maintaining a safe environment
2.	Communication
3.	Breathing
4.	Eating and drinking
5.	Elimination
6.	Washing and dressing
7.	Controlling temperature
8.	Mobilisation
9.	Working and playing
10.	Expressing sexuality
11.	Sleeping
12.	Death and dying

Source: Roper *et al.* (1999:19)

The Roper, Logan and Tierney Activities of Living nursing model was developed in Scotland by nursing academics Nancy Roper, Winifred Logan and Alison Tierney in the mid-1970s, and is widely used in the UK and Ireland (O'Connor 2002). It is used in conjunction with the Nursing Process. It takes into account the individuality of patients including their unique abilities, lifestyle and dependency level and where they are in their lifespan, and promotes individualised nursing rather than task-based nursing through the assessment, planning, implementation and evaluation of an individual's needs and care.

There are twelve activities identified in Table 1. Some of the activities are essential, such as breathing; and others enhance the quality of life, such as washing, dressing, working and playing; others are inevitable such as controlling body temperature, death and dying and elimination.

All twelve activities are influenced by five factors outlined in Table 2, including biological, psychological, socio-cultural, environmental and politico-economic, which are interlinked throughout all the activities. These prevent the nurse from focusing on 'the presenting problems' but allow the patient to be assessed and cared for in a holistic way, incorporating all twelve activities of living.

The information gained from the assessment of the activities of living is used in the planning stage of the Nursing Process to develop and plan goals of the care plan which ideally should be mutually agreed between the nurse, patient and the family. Care should be implemented according to the care plan and finally, evaluation of care establishes whether or not the goals of care have been achieved, or if they need to be reviewed.

The model recognises that depending where the individual is on the life-span scale (birth to old age), independence and dependence can be present, and acknowledges that while independence is valued, dependence should not affect or reduce the dignity of an individual (Roper *et al.*, 1999:34).

TABLE 2

Factors which influence the Activities of Living While these are individual factors they are interrelated.	
Biological	the anatomy and physiology of the human body
Psychological	cognitive development, intellectual aspects, emotional aspects
Sociocultural	spiritual, religious, cultural, community and ethical aspects; the role played within society (e.g. working/retired), status and relationships in society
Environmental	atmosphere, including light and sound, clothing and household environment
Politico-economic	the state, the law and the economy

Source: Roper *et al.*, (1999:42–51)

Table 3 links the activities of living with questions, triggers and ideas which can be used to assess and care for an individual. They help identify issues which may or may not be obvious on general observation. They identify areas which are actual problems as well as highlighting potential risks and allow the nurse to devise a care plan to suit the individual's needs. The questions are not exhaustive and not all questions apply to each patient.

TABLE 3

Activities of living triggers/questions/ideas	
Maintaining a safe environment	• What general safety issues are involved: brakes on bed, working equipment, fire exits etc.?
	• What is the cognitive ability of the individual?
	• Is the individual at risk of an accident?
	• Can the individual reach the call bell?
	• Are they safe to be left on their own?
	• What safety equipment does the individual require?
	• Is the patient an infection risk or at risk of infection?
	• Is there any risk associated with medication?
	• Does the individual have a history of falls, seizures, ear infections that may affect his or her balance?
	• Does he or she have any known allergies etc.?
Communication (including pain)	• Is the individual articulate, confused, cognitively impaired or do they have speech, visual problems etc.?
	• Is the individual hard of hearing, do they wear a hearing aid?
	• Does the individual understand/speak the language (English)?
	• Has the individual any visual signs of pain?
	• Do they express any pain verbally/non-verbally?
	• What is the pain score?
	• Does the individual have acute/chronic pain?
	• Can they describe the pain: pulsing, stabbing, burning, aching etc.?
	• Can they score the pain on a pain chart?
Mobility	• Is the individual independently mobile?
	• Do they use an aid such as walking stick, walking frame, crutches, wheelchair, motorised chair, suitable footwear etc.?
	• Does the individual have any illness which may affect their mobility such as chronic obstructive pulmonary disease, rheumatoid or osteo-arthritis etc.?
	• Does the individual need to use a hoist or support when moving?
	• Is their normal accommodation suitable for their mobility?

Controlling temperature	• Does the individual have a temperature?
	• Take all vital signs as required.
	• Are they pyrexic or hypothermic?
	• Do they have a history of fluctuating temperature?
	• Have they received medication to control their temperature?
	• Do they need extra blankets/covers etc.?
Breathing	• Is the individual short of breath now, when exercising or in the past?
	• Is the individual a smoker, non-smoker, ex-smoker?
	• Has the individual any pain when breathing?
	• What is the individual's pallor: red, pale, blue (cyanosis), grey?
	• Does the individual have any recent history of chest infections, lung diseases, asthma, etc.?
	• What are the individual's vital signs (blood pressure, respiration, pulse?
	• What are the rate, depth and rhythm of respirations and pulse?
Eating and drinking	• Has the individual any weight issues?
	• What weight are they?
	• Have they gained or lost weight recently?
	• Is the individual diabetic and if so are they insulin- or tablet-controlled?
	• Does the individual enjoy a good, normal appetite; what sort of food do they dislike etc.?
	• Has the individual any allergies to food or do they require a special diet, e.g. Kosher, Halal, low-sodium?
	• Does the individual have any mouth ulcers, dentures etc.? Do they need help when eating?
	• Do they drink enough each day, what types of drinks do they enjoy? If they consume alcohol, roughly how much per week do they consume?
	• Does the individual's fluid balance need to be monitored?

Elimination	• Does the individual have a regular bowel pattern?
	• Does the individual have a history of bowel disease?
	• Do they need medication/special diet to aid movement of bowels?
	• Does the individual have a stoma, if so where is it sited? How long has it been in situ? Does the individual experience any problems with it?
	• Does the individual have any history of urinary tract infections? if so is it a recurring problem, how is it being treated etc.?
	• Is the individual incontinent, do they experience urgency, have a catheter etc.?
	• Does the individual have any special equipment at home to help with elimination, such as bottles, adapted toilet etc.?
	• Is the colour or smell of the faeces or urine unusual? Do they contain blood?
Washing and dressing	• Does the individual need help washing, showering or bathing? Do they prefer a bath or a shower; do they have trouble getting in and out?
	• Do they use any special equipment in order to facilitate bathing, e.g. bath chairs, hoists etc.?
	• Are they able to dress themselves, do they have difficulty with buttons, laces etc.?
	• Do they use any aids to assist them when dressing?
Skin condition	• Assess the individual's skin and risk or presence of pressure sores. Use an assessment tool, e.g. Waterlow assessment scale.
	• Check if the individual has wounds or healthy, dry or papery skin.
	• Check if the individual has excessive sweating, any scratches, bruises, sores anywhere on their body and make a note of them.
	• Does the individual need assistance to turn or require equipment such as an air-flow bed etc.?
	• Are there any issues regarding oral hygiene?
	• Does the individual suffer from eczema, psoriasis etc. and does anything aggravate these conditions?
Working and playing	• What is the individual's job; are they retired, unemployed?
	• Does their health affect their job in any way?
	• Is the individual able to carry out their job without any problems?
	• What hobbies or interests does the individual have?
	• Are these affected by health issues, physical or mental health?

Sleep	• How many hours does the individual usually sleep?
	• What affects the individual's sleep pattern: noise, pain, anxiety etc.?
	• Is the individual's sleep pattern regular? Do they get up to go to the toilet during the night; if so how often?
	• Does the individual require any medication, alcoholic or milky drinks, to help them sleep?
Anxieties	• Does the individual have any worries or anxieties about being in hospital? (For example worry about leaving pets or family members alone whilst they are in hospital, or they might be frightened about the hospital environment and what is going to happen to them.)
	• Does the individual need to be introduced to the layout of the ward, or is it necessary to explain why they are in hospital and what treatment they may expect?
	• Is it necessary to demonstrate to the individual how to use the nurse call system; do they need to be informed about the procedure for ordering meals etc.?
	• Does the individual need reassurance or to be helped to feel more comfortable both physically and emotionally?
Expressing sexuality	• Are there any health-related issues linked to individual's sexuality?
	• What are the individual's preferences regarding make-up, clothes etc.; would it be appropriate for the individual to dress each day etc.?
	• Are there any issues such as low self esteem or decreased sexual activity related to alteration of the body as a result of surgery, e.g. mastectomy, pregnancy, diet, heart attack etc.?
	• Privacy/dignity issues, e.g. patient confused and throwing off clothes?
Death and dying	• Is the individual receiving palliative care?
	• Has the individual any anxieties or concerns about death and dying?
	• Does the individual have religious preferences?
	• Has there been a recent bereavement?
	• What physical care is required: dry mouth, regular turning, special bed etc.?
	• Is there a need for counselling, pastoral care etc.?
	• Are there any special religious practices that need to be carried out when the person dies, e.g. Muslim, Jewish?

It may not always be appropriate or necessary to ask the individual all the questions above due to condition, cognitive ability or awareness. In some areas different policies apply regarding information required, at other times professional judgement will be used to decide which questions need to be prioritised.

ACTIVITY

Case study

Tom is an 82-year-old widowed man who lives alone in a two-storey semi-detached house and has two sons who live locally. He is admitted to your hospital following an unexplained fall. He has shortness of breath on admission and has difficulty mobilising. Tom has pain on movement and appears agitated and is disorientated as to time and place. Tom is very thin and has an unkempt appearance on admission.

Use the case study above or develop your own case study on a potential client or an elderly person you know and use Table 3 to identify appropriate questions which would determine Tom's potential and actual problems and assist you to assess Tom.

Revision

1. Discuss what is meant by a theory of nursing, a concept and a model of nursing.

2. Make notes to explain the difference between a theory of nursing and a model of nursing.

3. What are the three basic components of a model of nursing?

4. Discuss how the application of models to practice influences the activity of the nurse and the experience for the patient or client.

5. Outline the main features of the Roy and Orem models of nursing.

6. What does the Roper, Logan and Tierney nursing model suggest about the person, environment, health and nursing?

7. Draw a mind map to name the twelve activities of living and expand on each activity using Table 3.

8. Identify five factors which influence the activities of living.

9. Identify actual and potential problems from the needs identified above.

References

Aggleton, P. and Chalmers, H., *Nursing Models and the Nursing Process*, 2nd ed., London: Macmillan 1992.

Chinn, P. and Kramer, M., *Integrated Knowledge Development in Nursing*, St Louis: C. V. Mosby 2004.

Fawcett, J., *Analysis and Evaluation of Conceptual Models of Nursing*, 3rd ed., Philadelphia: F. A. Davis 1995.

Fawcett, J., 'The metaparadigm of nursing: current status and future refinements' in *Journal of Nursing Scholarship* 16:3 (1984), 84–7.

Girot, E., 'Discussing nursing theory', *Senior Nurse* 10(6) (1990), 16–19.

Hodgson, R., 'A nursing muse', *British Journal of Nursing* 1:7 (1992), 330–33.

Kenny, T., 'Nursing models fail in practice', *British Journal of Nursing* 2 (1993), 133–36.

Miller, A., 'Models in nursing', *Nursing Times* 80:51 (1984), 13.

Murphy, F. *et al.*, 'Nursing models and contemporary nursing 1: their development, uses and limitations', *Nursing Times* 106:23, available at www.nursingtimes.net/nursing-practice/clinical-zones/practice-nursing/nursing-models-and-contemporary-nursing-1-their-development-uses-and-limitations-/5015918.article (2010) (accessed 1/8/13).

O'Connor, M., 'Using the Roper, Logan and Tierney model in a neonatal ICU' available at www.nursingtimes.net/nursing-practice/clinical-zones/childrens-nursing/using-the-roper-logan-and-tierney-model-in-a-neonatal-icu/199604.article (2002) (accessed 1/8/13)

Parker, M. and Smith, M., *Nursing Theories and Nursing Practice*, 3rd ed., Philadelphia: F. A. Davis 2010.

Pearson, A. *et al.*, *Nursing Models for Practice*, 2nd ed., Oxford: Butterworth-Heinemann 1996.

Roper, N. *et al.*, *The Elements of Nursing: A Model of Nursing Based on a Model of Living*, 4th ed., London: Churchill Livingstone 1999.

Roper, N. *et al.*, *The Roper, Logan, Tierney Model of Nursing Based on Activities of Living*, London: Churchill Livingstone 2005.

Empathic Behaviour of the Care Worker

At the end of this chapter the learner should be able to:

- describe what is meant by empathic behaviour
- outline the difference between sympathy, compassion and empathy
- discuss the different factors that the care worker needs to consider when building an empathic relationship in nursing
- identify the role of advocacy in empathic behaviour
- define advocacy
- name four different types of advocacy
- identify four skills required for effective advocacy
- define communication
- outline the interrelationship between interpersonal skills and effective communication
- identify what is involved in skilful interpersonal behaviour
- identify the 'five i's' in the effective communication framework
- explain four barriers to communication and interaction with patients

Empathic behaviour of the care worker

Empathic behaviour of the care worker involves a number of components, such as empathy which is a common and regularly debated topic in the nursing literature; advocacy, which may be required by an individual, group or family; communication, personal and interpersonal skills and interview techniques and skills which are essential in all aspects of nursing. While interview techniques and skills related to obtaining information are discussed in Chapter 4 on the Nursing Process, the other components identified on page 43 are discussed in this chapter.

Empathy

Dinkins (2011) suggests that empathy is one of the basic building blocks of ethics and ethical conduct toward others. Without empathy it is difficult for any of us to understand the needs and wants of others so that they are treated with respect and generosity and it would be almost impossible to demonstrate and practise honesty, goodness, morality or any other virtue in our day-to-day relations with them.

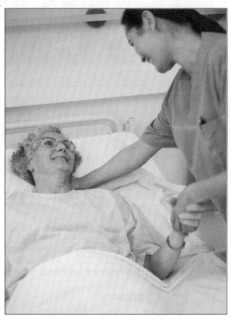

When trying to empathise with fellow humans, it is necessary to observe verbal signs and body language as well as an individual's external appearance and signs such as a smile, a heavy sigh or a haggard appearance to gauge how they feel. However, empathy also involves trying to share and understand something internal, for example another's feelings, instincts, worries or desires. It can be difficult to decode the external and internal signs that lead to empathic understanding. If an individual has not experienced an event, or has had a different experience of the same event, or has little life experience, there can be difficulties in empathising.

Sometimes empathy is confused with sympathy and compassion, as these terms are commonly used in nursing. However, they have different meanings, as outlined in Table 1.

TABLE 1: DEFINITION OF TERMS

Sympathy	the verbal and nonverbal expression of sorrow or dismay (Morse *et al.*, 1992)
Compassion	active participation in another individual's suffering (Schantz, 2007)
Empathy	an understanding not only of the other's beliefs, values and ideas but also the significance that their situation has for them, and their associated feelings (Rogers, 1951)

(Chowdhry, 2010)

What is empathy in nursing?

The term empathy has its basis in psychology and is considered to play an important part in the counselling relationship; however, it is acknowledged that the boundaries of the everyday counselling relationship will vary from that of the nurse–patient relationship. According to von Dietze and Orb (2000), the focus of empathy is intellectual or professional and this allows nurses to remain detached from their patients.

Within counselling literature, empathy is defined as having the capacity to identify and understand another individual's emotions and feelings (Chowdhry, 2010). Empathy within the nursing relationship is defined as a human trait, a professional state, a communication process, caring, and a special relationship (Yu and Kirk, 2008). The value of empathy for the nurse–patient relationship is that it is thought to allow understanding not only of another individual's beliefs, values and ideas but also the significance that their situation has for them, and their associated feelings.

Chowdhry (2010) cites Rogers (1951) who suggests that in counselling sessions empathy forms part of the set of 'core conditions' along with congruence (being genuine and transparent) and unconditional positive regard (being non-judgemental) which ultimately enables the client to become less judgemental of themselves and more consistent, and empowers and aids them to find their own way forward through life's problems.

Yu and Kirk (2008) suggest that interest in the role of empathy within the nurse–patient relationship has been growing over the past few decades and is often considered to be a vital component of a good standard of therapeutic care (Reynolds *et al.*, 1999). However there is another side to empathy in nursing which needs to be highlighted. Patients trust nurses who are empathic towards them as they feel that the nurse cares about them (Määttä, 2006). It is important to be aware that in the relationship between the nurse and the patient, generally the patient is more vulnerable (Sellman, 2007). The trust that is potentially created by the empathic relationship may mean that the patient discloses information that, in any other situation, they might not disclose; this type of relationship could lead to the sharing of deeply personal information that could be used in a variety of ways.

While the nurse in the empathic relationship may not be deliberately trying to exploit their patient they need to be aware of professional boundaries, patient empowerment and confidentiality rights. In the healthcare sector confidentiality refers to the appropriate protection of the personal and private details of clients' situations or conditions. It is not about keeping a secret, but about sharing, transmitting and storing the information in an appropriate manner (Walsh *et al.*, 2005). The boundaries of confidentiality and professionalism are subjective and patients may think that something they say to a nurse or doctor they trust and with whom they have an empathic relationship will automatically be kept secret, however this may not be the view of the nurse or doctor (Jenkins, 2005). If the information is used in the wrong context it may lead to misunderstandings and possible lack of empowerment for the patient. This means that consent should be gained and it should be clearly identified whether the patient wishes to have their personal feelings documented or shared with the healthcare team.

It is vital when empathising or building an empathic relationship with a patient that the nurse understands the roles played by consent, confidentiality, empowerment and nurse advocacy.

Advocacy

The *Scope of Nursing and Midwifery Practice Framework* (2000) considers values which should underpin nursing practice. It suggests that nursing practice involves advocacy for the individual patient/client and for their family. It also involves advocacy on behalf of nursing within the organisational and management structures within which it is delivered (An Bord Altranais, 2000). It is essential that nurses who are on the frontline caring for patients develop and use advocacy skills to address workplace concerns, promote positive work environments, and advocate for the profession (Tomajan, 2012).

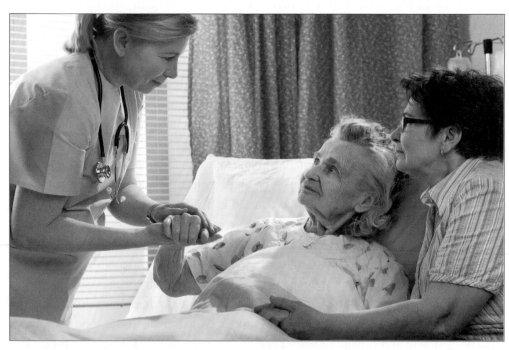

As defined by Inclusion Ireland, advocacy is 'taking action to enable people to express what they want, secure their rights, represent their interests, and obtain services they need. Advocates and advocacy services work in partnership with the people they support and take their side. Advocacy promotes social inclusion, equality, and social justice.'

Types of advocacy

Public policy advocacy

Public policy advocacy is carried out by organisations which campaign for changes to laws, policies and services in respect of people who are vulnerable, for example people with intellectual disabilities. They make submissions to government and public bodies, participate on working groups and committees, organise campaigns and speak out on behalf of people with particular needs.

Representative advocacy

Representative advocacy is support provided by a paid advocate to an individual to have their voice heard in respect of a particular issue. This is sometimes called professional or independent advocacy.

Self-advocacy

Self-advocacy is when a person speaks up for themselves, alone or as part of a group.

Parent advocacy

Parent advocacy is about parents acting as advocates for their children.

Peer advocacy

Peer advocacy is when a person with a shared experience supports another person to have their voice heard.

Citizen advocacy

Advocacy can also be provided in a non-paid capacity. The main difference between citizen advocacy and representative advocacy is that the relationship in citizen advocacy is long-term and the advocate's time is given freely.

Advocacy in nursing

The Royal College of Nursing (1992) defined advocacy as 'a process of acting for, or on behalf of someone who is unable to do so for themselves'. Advocacy is recognised as a role in nursing, and it has been suggested that advocacy in nursing may differ from the legal type of advocacy where a person is asked or allocated to be an advocate. Vaartio (2006) reports that nursing advocacy is expressed by voicing responsiveness, and includes an acknowledged professional responsibility for and active involvement in supporting patients' needs and wishes.

Nurses are not invited by patients to care for them, but are in a privileged relationship that confers trust upon the nurse and assumes that they will act in the interests of the patient, making a good assessment of needs. Not all patients want the nurse to act as their advocate. Evidence suggests that the nature and context of relationships plays a significant role in influencing the enactment of advocacy (MacDonald, 2007). Nurses should, therefore, not presume to be advocates of patients, yet should always act in patients' best interests (Bennett, 1999). Though it may be considered that the patient needs support, for example when talking to medical staff, it is important to identify whether a patient has the confidence or ability do this rather than for the nurse to take over and talk on the patient's behalf when the patient could speak for themselves, as advocacy must be a need expressed by the patient, not perceived by the nurse. The nurse, in the role of advocate, should not try to undermine the autonomy of the patient.

Skills required for advocacy

Tomajan (2012) suggests the following skills are required for effective advocacy.

Communication

Advocates need to communicate openly and concisely and to ensure the message is appropriate for both the situation and the intended audience. It is important to understand the client's objective. Advocates must be comfortable with all communication formats, such as verbal, written and electronic formats. Effective listening is vital, as is the ability to engage in oral discussion in a clear and concise, factual manner.

Influence others to action

The ability to influence others to action involves altering or changing an individual's or group's ideas, beliefs or actions and is essential to the advocacy process. Influence is built on the credibility, competence and trustworthiness of the advocate.

Problem-solving

Patience and a good sense of timing are necessary in order to achieve a successful outcome. Successful advocacy interventions are achieved through negotiation, collaboration, and compromise; they may require a series of actions over time in order to achieve an outcome.

Collaboration

The advocate must have the ability to work with and build relationships with people in all roles and identify who is the best person to assist with the advocacy issues in question.

ACTIVITY

Using role play, in pairs outline a situation where a patient has a particular issue and the nurse identifies that there is a problem. As an advocate and a person in an empathic relationship discuss the skills required to assist the individual and the factors that need to be kept in mind when a client or patient is discussing personal feelings and disclosing information.

Communication and interpersonal skills

The Health Information and Quality Authority (HIQA) in the *National Standards for Safer Better Healthcare* (2012) concluded that the health service provided to all individuals should be person-centred. HIQA highlights the need for service providers to communicate in a manner that supports the development of a relationship based 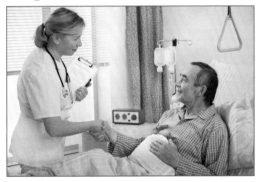 on trust. They recommend good communication and the provision of adequate information to ensure that service users can make informed decisions about their care, including the opportunity to give or refuse consent to treatment.

Communication with service users in a manner that respects their dignity and privacy is essential to an effective service. Walsh *et al.* (2005) maintain that effective care workers have very good communication skills and good interpersonal skills, including the ability to listen, to establish and maintain relationships, to observe and respond to nonverbal communication, as well as an awareness of the various technologies which are available to promote communication.

Communication is considered a basic tool in healthcare relationships and the effectiveness of the communication will be determined by the quality of the communication (Bach and Grant, 2009). The interrelationship between communication and interpersonal skills, the importance of these concepts in nursing and how, when used in a structured, effective way, they can support a carer to behave in an empathic manner, is discussed below.

The interrelationship between communication and interpersonal skills

Bach and Grant (2009) define communication as an exchange of information between people by means of speaking, writing or using a common system of signs or behaviour.

The term 'interpersonal' describes the connection between two or more people or groups and their involvement with one another, especially as regards the way they behave towards and feel about one another (Bach and Grant, 2009).

Communication has been described as a complex process that involves passing a message intentionally or unintentionally between two people (Redfern and Ross, 2006).

The simple model outlined below suggests four components of good communication.

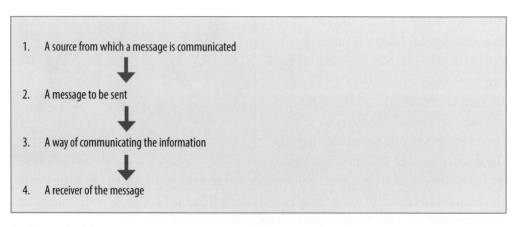

At the end of these stages a message is usually returned to the source creating an ongoing process. However there are times when this process is not possible or is interrupted due to cognitive ability, physical or emotional health, environment or resources. Webb (2011) suggests effective communication relies a great deal on the skills of the message sender and the ability of the receiver to interpret what is being communicated. These aspects of communication represent the interpersonal skills of a good communicator. They help build an empathic relationship as well as providing tools for the carer who needs to advocate for a patient. The skilled communicator presents information in a clear and concise manner and demonstrates good listening skills. In addition, a skilled communicator is aware of and makes allowances for barriers to communication, such as cultural differences, the emotional and cognitive states of individuals, as well as external distractions.

Michael Argyle (1983, in Webb, 2011) suggests that skilful interpersonal behaviour includes the following:

- perception of others' reactions, for example the communicator is in tune with the other person's behaviour and knows when an individual is showing signs of understanding or misunderstanding

- attention to feedback and corrective action and identification of the type of response needed, for example an encouraging remark or the use of open-ended questions to probe for more information

- awareness of the right timing of social responses, knowing when to speak or interpret and when to remain silent and listen

- self-awareness and the ability to use this self-knowledge to present oneself to the other; this gives the other feedback about who the communicator is and therefore how to interpret and respond to them. For instance, sitting in a forward-leaning position assures the other that they are being listened to

- 'rewardingness': the ability to engage the other in the communication and know how to reward communication behaviour, for instance, using nods, smiles and eye contact to encourage someone to talk about themselves

These are just some interpersonal skills required for effective communication and interaction with patients. In summary, interpersonal skills are skills that allow people to communicate effectively with each other. Good interpersonal skills help develop social skills and lead to effective communication using appropriate techniques. Many of these skills can be learned and developed through practice and through personal development by improving self-awareness and awareness and understanding of other people and their cognitive and emotional states.

> ### ACTIVITY
>
> Using role play, identify a messenger and a receiver and have the messenger tell a story to the receiver. When completed identify the interpersonal skills used as outlined above and reflect on the outcome for both parties.
>
> Then change roles and have the messenger tell a story while the receiver ignores the use of these skills. Reflect on how both of you feel about the encounter in this situation.

Communication and interpersonal skills in nursing

Harrison and Hart (2006) and Northouse and Northouse (2004) outline the range of communication skills available to health professionals. Nurses can facilitate successful and therapeutic patient contact through questioning, listening, summarising, reflecting, paraphrasing and closure. Nurses use these skills routinely to gather information; reassure; facilitate patient expression; establish attitudes, views and opinions; encourage critical thinking; reduce anxiety; facilitate liaison with other disciplines and promote continuity in patient care (Berry, 2007 and Bury, 2005).

Interpersonal skills while not exclusive to nursing are necessary to develop relationships and effectively communicate with colleagues, team members, patients, clients and staff. Good communication in the nurse–patient encounter is itself a beneficial and therapeutic intervention as well as being necessary to maintain good standards of care, and may be as important as other care or treatment. Dougherty and Lister (2007) identified potential reduction of the effects of pain and increased recovery rates when patients were provided with additional information/communication about their condition, diagnosis, prognosis, required care and treatment.

Framework for effective communication skills

Hamilton and Martin (2007) illustrate a framework for effective communication skills practice called 'the five i's' which is summarised in Table 2. These five factors require the use of a variety of interpersonal skills in order to identify whether communication and interaction is successful or needs to be reviewed.

TABLE 2: THE FIVE I'S

1	**INTERACT** with the patient
2	Identify the **INTENTION** of the interaction
3	Decide on the **INTERVENTION** to be used for the interaction
4	Assess the **IMPACT** of the intervention(s)
5	Evaluate the **IMPLICATIONS** of the subsequent information obtained and then act accordingly

1. Interact

Nurses should use the full range of communication skills to interact with patients in order to make it clear to patients that practitioners are there to help as much as they possibly can, both physically and psychologically, in view of the patient's present state of health. Patients must be given time and space to express their fears, anxieties, concerns or worries and nurses must demonstrate a willingness to engage, interact and communicate.

2. Intention

Nurses should establish what the intentions of the interaction are. Communication skills are the lifeblood of any interaction, whether personal, professional, social or otherwise, but structure or goals must be present in order to maximise the likelihood of effective interaction (Murray *et al.*, 2006).

3. Interventions

Nurses also need to decide on the most appropriate interventions. These interventions may be verbal or nonverbal and may take a physical or psychological form depending on the overall aim and purpose of the interaction, for example administering medication; carrying out vital signs observations; assisting an elderly person with their activities of daily living or reassuring an anxious patient using communication skills.

4. Impact of interventions

Nurses should then assess and reflect on the impact of the selected interventions. Have they met their goals? Did the selected intervention or interventions work? If not, why not? What could be done differently next time to maximise the likelihood of a successful interaction?

5. *Implications*

The final step is to evaluate the implications of the interaction for professionals and patients. For example, obtaining information from a patient on admission during an assessment-type interview is appropriate but depending on the information received other members of the multidisciplinary team may need to be involved in the patient's care and treatment.

Barriers to communication and interaction with patients

Bach and Grant (2009) discussed the many complexities present in the healthcare environment that are often similar to those in our everyday lives but are heightened by factors such as healthcare policy, environment, levels of responsibility, cultural and language difficulties, physical illness and discomfort, anxiety, sadness and fear. It is evident that the healthcare environment presents an even more complicated set of circumstances to deal with than when we communicate or interact with family or friends.

Communication and healthcare interactions are often delivered in demanding and stressful circumstances, which inevitably leads to further demands on the carer's abilities to communicate effectively. Bach and Grant (2009) suggest that, while qualified nurses often rate their own communication skills as high, patients report less satisfaction and maintain that communication could be improved. In addition, there is evidence that some nurses stereotype patient groups (Timmins, 2007). Therefore it is important that those in the caring professions take time to become aware of themselves and their abilities and learn in more detail about communicating in healthcare settings in order to communicate and interact effectively and provide care in an empathic manner.

Revision

1. Write down what you understand by empathic behaviour.
2. Identify the differences between sympathy, compassion and empathy.
3. Discuss the different factors that the care worker needs to consider when building an empathic relationship in nursing.
4. Identify the role of advocacy in empathic behaviour.
5. Define advocacy.
6. Name and outline four different types of advocacy.

7. Using a mind map, identify four skills required for effective advocacy.
8. Define communication.
9. In pairs, discuss the interrelationship between interpersonal skills and effective communication.
10. Identify what is involved in skilful interpersonal behaviour.
11. Name the 'five i's' in the effective communication framework.
12. Identify and explain four barriers to communication and interaction with patients.

References

An Bord Altranais, *Scope of Nursing and Midwifery Practice Framework*, Dublin: An Bord Altranais 2000.

Bach, S. and Grant, A., *Communication and Interpersonal Skills for Nurses*, Exeter: Learning Matters 2009.

Bennett, O., 'Advocacy in nursing', *Nursing Standard* 14:11 (1999), 40–41.

Berry, D., *Healthcare Communication: Theory and Practice*, London: Open University Press 2007.

Bury, M., *Health and Illness*, UK: Blackwell Scientific Publications 2005.

Chowdhry, S., 'Exploring the concept of empathy in nursing: can it lead to abuse of patient trust?', *Nursing Times* 106 (2010), 42.

Dinkins, C., 'Ethics: beyond patient care: practicing empathy in the workplace', *The Online Journal of Issues in Nursing* 16:2 (2011).

Dougherty, L. and Lister, S., eds, *The Royal Marsden Hospital Manual of Clinical Nursing Procedures*, London: Blackwell Publishing 2007.

Hamilton, S. J. and Martin, D. J., 'A framework for effective communication skills', *Nursing Times* 103:48 (2007), 30–31.

Harrison, A. and Hart, C. *Mental Health Care for Nurses: Applying Mental Health Skills in the General Hospital*, London: Blackwell Publishing 2006.

Health Information and Quality Authority, *National Standards for Safer Better Healthcare*, Dublin: HIQA 2012.

Inclusion Ireland, 'Advocacy' available at http://www.inclusionireland.ie/content/page/advocacy (accessed 2/9/13)

Jenkins, G., 'A qualitative study of women's views on medical confidentiality', *Journal of Medical Ethics* 31:9 (2005), 499–504.

Määttä, S. M., 'Closeness and distance in the nurse–patient relation: the relevance of Edith Stein's concept of empathy', *Nursing Philosophy* 7 (2006), 3–10.

MacDonald, H., 'Relational ethics and advocacy in nursing: literature review', *Journal of Advanced Nursing* 57:2 (2007), 119–26.

Murray, K. *et al.*, 'Effective communication and its delivery in midwifery practice', *The Practising Midwife* 9:4 (2006), 24–6.

Northouse, L. L. and Northouse, P. G., *Health Communication: Strategies for Health Professionals*, London: Prentice Hall 2004.

Redfern, S. and Ross, F., *Nursing Older People*, 4th ed., London: Churchill Livingstone 2006.

Reynolds, W. J. *et al.*, 'Empathy has not been measured in clients' terms or effectively taught: a review of the literature', *Journal of Advanced Nursing* 30:5 (1999), 1177–85.

Royal College of Nursing, *Issues in Nursing and Health: Advocacy and the Nurse*, London, RCN 1992.

Sellman, D. 'Trusting patients, trusting nurses', *Nursing Philosophy* 8 (2007), 28–36.

Timmins, F., 'Communication skills: revisiting the fundamentals', *Nurse Prescribing* 5 (2007), 395–9.

Tomajan, K., 'Advocating for Nurses and Nursing', *The Online Journal of Issues in Nursing* 17:1 (2012).

Vaartio, H. *et al.,* 'Nursing advocacy: how is it defined by patients and nurses, what does it involve and how is it experienced?', *Scandinavian Journal of Caring Sciences* 20:3 (2006), 282–92.

von Dietze, E. V. and Orb, A. 'Compassionate care: a moral dimension in nursing', *Nursing Inquiry* 7:3 (2000), 166–74.

Walsh, M. *et al.*, *Health and Social Care*, London: Collins 2005.

Webb, L. *Nursing: Communication Skills in Practice*, Oxford: Oxford University Press 2011.

Yu, J. and Kirk, M., 'Measurement of empathy in nursing research: systematic review', *Journal of Advanced Nursing* 64:5 (2008), 440–54.

Medical Terminology and Abbreviations

At the end of this chapter the learner should be able to:

- explain commonly used nursing and medical terminology, as well as:
  - ▸ show knowledge of the structure of medical words
  - ▸ make connections between commonly used terms in different situations
  - ▸ explain commonly used nursing and medical abbreviations
  - ▸ demonstrate knowledge and understanding of uses and conditions of usage

Medical terminology

Many medical terms originate from ancient Greece and Rome. They include terms to describe body systems, body organs and their functions. An understanding of medical terms helps nurses, doctors and other healthcare professionals to communicate clearly with each other. A nurse's dictionary is an essential purchase for every nurse in training.

Correct spelling is vitally important. In medical records incorrect spelling could change the meaning of a word or term and affect the care of a patient.

There are three components to each medical word:

1. roots/combining forms
2. prefixes
3. suffixes

Roots

A word root is the basic foundation of a word which gives its general meaning. Roots are usually combined using a vowel (referred to as a combining form – *i* or *o* are the most commonly used), for example:

cardi- (heart)

pulmon- (lungs)

haemat- (blood)

Prefixes

Prefixes are added to the beginning of a word root to change its meaning or create a new word, for example:

tachy- (fast/rapid), e.g. tachycardia

brady- (slow), e.g. bradycardia

hypo- (low), e.g. hypothermia

hyper- (high), e.g. hyperthermia

pre- (before), e.g. pre-operation

post- (after), e.g. post-operation

Suffixes

Suffixes are placed at the end of a word to tell us what is happening to a particular body part, for example:

-itis, e.g. appendicitis (inflammation of appendix)

-logy, e.g. pathology (study of disease and its effects)

-ior, e.g. posterior (back or behind)

(Henderson and Dorsey, 2009)

ACTIVITY

Using a medical or nursing dictionary, find the definitions of the following commonly used medical terms:

Afferent	Bronchitis
Anaemia	Carcinoma
Anterior	Cardiac
Arteriosclerosis	Cholecystitis
Bradycardia	Dehydration

Diarrhoea	Myocardium
Dysmenorrhoea	Neonate
Dyspnoea	Neoplasm
Dysuria	Nephron
Efferent	Nephrosis
Emphysema	Oedema
Endocrine	Oliguria
Gastroenteritis	Ophthalmic
Gastrointestinal	Pathogen
Gene	Physiology
Genetic	Pneumothorax
Haematuria	Polyuria
Haemoglobin	Sensory
Hepatic	Sigmoid
Hydrocephalus	Sublingual
Hypertrophy	Tachycardia
Hypotension	Thrombosis
Intracranial	Vasoconstriction
Microbe	

Abbreviations

Full text is always preferable to abbreviations. If you use abbreviations they should be from an approved list from the healthcare facility or from the *Code of Practice for Healthcare Records Management* (HSE, 2010). The list should be reviewed periodically and updated accordingly (ABA, 2002).

Rules for using abbreviations

Only use abbreviations from the approved list. If there is no abbreviation for the term you wish to use you must write it in full followed by your own abbreviation in brackets, and ensure the term is written both in full and abbreviated in brackets on every page it is used.

All abbreviations must be in capital letters.

Shortening of a word is acceptable if it is on the list. Use a capital letter at the start of the word and finish with a full stop (HSE, 2011).

Abbreviations should never be used in the following situations or on the following documents:

1. Instructions regarding the resuscitation status of a patient. If a patient is not for active measures this must be written in full; do not write 'DNR' (Do Not Resuscitate)

2. Drug names

3. R and L must be written as 'right' and 'left'

4. +++, <, > should be avoided unless part of a grading system, as in urinalysis results

5. Pos. and Neg. should be used instead of -ve and +ve

6. Service user's name should be written in full

7. Transfer documents

8. Discharge letters

9. Referral letters

10. Consent forms

11. Death certificates

12. Prescription letters

13. Letters going to an external facility or healthcare provider
    (HSE, 2011)

The most recent list of approved abbreviations is available from http://www.hse.ie/eng/services/Publications/services/Hospitals/NHO_Code_of_Practice_for_Healthcare_Records_Management_Version_2_0.pdf.

The following are commonly used abbreviations you may come across on work placement; they have been taken from *NHO Code of Practice for Healthcare Record Management* (HSE, 2010):

A

ABC	Airway breathing circulation
Abd.	Abdominal
AD	Alzheimer's Disease
ADL	Activities of daily living
Adm.	Admission/admitted
ADON/M	Assistant Director of Midwifery/Nursing
AIDS	Acquired immune deficiency syndrome
a.m.	Morning before twelve
Anaes.	Anaesthetic
ANP	Advanced Nurse Practitioner
Ant.	Anterior
APH	Ante partum haemorrhage
Approx.	Approximately
Appt.	Appointment
ASAP	As soon as possible
Ass.	Assistance
Ausc.	Auscultation
Ax.	Assessment

B

Ba. Enema	Barium enema
BBA	Born before admission/arrival
BC	Blood cultures
b.d./b.i.d.	Twice daily
BG	Blood glucose/blood gases
BGL	Blood glucose level

BMI	Body mass index		Cx.	Cervix
BMR	Basal metabolic rate		CxR	Chest x-Ray
BNO	Bowels not open			

D

BO	Bowels opened
BOS	Base of support
BP	Blood pressure
BPM	Beats per minute
Bx.	Biopsy

C

Ca.	Carcinoma
CAD	Coronary artery disease
cc	Copied to
CCF	Congestive cardiac failure
CCU	Coronary Care unit
Chemo	Chemotherapy
CHO	Carbohydrate
Chol.	Cholesterol
CLD	Chronic lung disease
cm	Centimetre
CMM 1,2,3	Clinical Midwife Manager 1,2,3
CNM 1,2,3	Clinical Nurse Manager 1,2,3
CNS	Central nervous system
CO_2	Carbon dioxide
CO	Complaining of
COLD	Chronic obstructive lung disease
Conc.	Concentration
Cons.	Consultant
Cont'd.	Continued
COPD	Chronic obstructive pulmonary disease
CRF	Chronic renal failure
CandS	Culture and Sensitivity
CS	Caesarean section
CSE	Combined spinal epidural
CSF	Cerebrospinal fluid
CSU	Catheter specimen of urine
CT	Computerised tomography
CV	Cardiovascular
CVA	Cerebrovascular accident
CVL	Central venous line
CVP	Central venous pressure
CVS	Cardiovascular system

DBE	Deep breathing exercises
DandC	Dilatation and curettage
Dc.	Discharge
Defib.	Defibrillation
Dept.	Department
DM	Diabetes mellitus
DNA	Did not attend
DOA	Dead on arrival
DOB	Date of birth
DOM/N	Director of Midwifery/ Nursing
DPM	Drops per minute
Dr.	Doctor
DTs	Delirium tremens
DandV	Diarrhoea and vomiting
DVT	Deep vein thrombosis
DW	Discussed with
Dx/	Diagnosis

E

EA	Elective admission
EBL	Estimated blood loss
ECg	Electrocardiogram
ECHO	Echocardiogram
E. Coli	*Escherichia coli*
ECT	Electroconvulsive therapy
ED	Emergency department
EDD	Estimated date of delivery
e.g.	For example
Enc.	Enclosed
ENT	Ear nose and throat
Est. Req.	Estimated requirements
EUA	Examination under anaesthetic

F

FB	Foreign body
FBC	Full blood count
FBS	Fasting blood sugar
Fe	Iron
FFP	Fresh frozen plasma

FH	Foetal heart
FHHR	Foetal heart heard and regular
FMF	Foetal movement felt
FOB	Faecal occult blood
FU	Follow up
FWB	Full weight bearing

G

g	gram
GA	General anaesthetic
GBS	Group B *Streptococcus*
GCS	Glasgow coma scale
gest.	Gestation
GF	Gluten-free
GandH	Group and hold
GI	Gastro-intestinal
GIT	Gastro-intestinal tract
GO	Gastro-oesophageal
GORD	Gastro-oesophageal reflux disorder/disease
GP	General Practitioner
GTT	Glucose tolerance test
GU	Genito-urinary
GXM	Group and cross match

H

H	Hour
Haem.	Haematology
Hams.	Hamstrings
Hb	Haemoglobin
HC	Head circumference
HCA	Home care assistant
HDu	High dependency unit
Hep. A/B/C	Hepatitis A/B/C
HH	Home help
HI	Head injury
HIV	Human immunodeficiency virus
HR	Heart rate
HRT	Hormone replacement therapy
HSE	Health Service Executive
Ht.	Height
HTN	Hypertension
HV	Home visit

HVS	High vaginal swab
Hx.	History

I

ICU	Intensive care unit
IandD	Incision and drainage
ID	Infectious disease
i.e.	that is
Ig	Immunoglobulin
IHD	Ischaemic heart disease
IHF	Irish Heart Foundation
IM	Intramuscular
Imp.	Impression
Incl.	Including/included
Ind.	Independent
Inf.	Inferior
Info.	Information
In Pt.	In-patient
INR	International normalised ratio
ITT	Insulin tolerance test
ITU	Intensive therapy unit
IU	International unit
IUD	Intrauterine contraceptive device
IV	Intravenous
IVI	Intravenous infusion
IWA	Irish Wheelchair Association
Ix.	Investigation

K

k+	Potassium
kcal	kilocalorie
kCL	Potassium chloride
kg.	kilogram
kJ	kilojoules

L

L	Litre
LA	Local anaesthetic
Lab.	Laboratory
Lat.	Lateral
lbs.	Pounds weight
LFTs	Liver function tests
LIF	Left iliac fossa
LIH	Left inguinal hernia

LOC	Loss of consciousness
LP	Lumbar puncture
LSCS	Lower segment caesarean section
LTC	Long-term care
LTM	Long-term memory
LVF	Left ventricular failure
Ly.	Lying

M

Mane	Morning
MAU	Medical assessment/admission unit
Max.	Maximum
MDT	Multidisciplinary team
Meds.	Medication
Mets.	Metastases
mg	millligram
Mg2+	Magnesium
MI	Myocardial infarction
Micro.	Microbiology
Min.	Minimum
Mins.	Minute
mL	millilitre
mm	millimetre
mmHg	millimetres of mercury
mmol	millimole
MMR	Measles, mumps, rubella
MND	Motor neurone disease
Mob.	Mobility/mobilising
MRI	Magnetic resonance imaging
MROP	Manual removal of placenta
MRSA	Methicillin resistant *Staphylococcus aureus*
MS	Multiple sclerosis
Msg.	Message
MSSA	Methicillin sensitive *Staphylococcus aureus*
MSU	Midstream specimen of urine

N

N_2O	Nitrous oxide
NA	Not applicable
Na+	Sodium
NaCL	Sodium chloride

NAD	No abnormality detected
NB	*Nota bene* (important)
Neg.	Negative
Neuro.	Neurological
NFA	No fixed abode
NFR	Not for resuscitation
Ng	Naso-gastric
NH	Nursing home
NKA	No known allergies
NkDA	No known drug allergies
No.	Number
Nocte	Night
NOF	Neck of femur
NOK	Next of kin
NP	New patient
NPO	Nil per oral
NPU	Not passed urine
NSAID	Non-steroidal anti-inflammatory drug(s)
NandV	Nausea and vomiting
NWB	Non-weight bearing

O

O_2	Oxygen
OA	Osteoarthritis
OAusc.	On auscultation
Obj.	Objective
Obs.	Observations
Occ.	Occasional
OD	Overdose
OE	On examination
Onc.	Oncology
OP	Outpatient
OPD	Outpatient department
Ortho.	Orthopaedics
OT	Occupational therapy/therapist

P

Paeds.	Paediatrics
PCA	Patient controlled analgesia
PE	Pulmonary embolus/embolism
PEARL	Pupils equal and reacting to light
PHN	Public health nurse

Physio.	Physiotherapist/physiotherapy		RIF	Right iliac fossa
PID	Pelvic inflammatory disease		RIP	Rest in peace/deceased
PKU	Phenylketonuria		RLQ	Right lower quadrant
PLTS	Platelets		RM	Registered midwife
p.m.	Afternoon		RO	Removal of
PMHx.	Past medical history		RR	Respiratory/respiration rate
PO	Per oral		RT	Radiotherapy
POP	Plaster of paris		RTA	Road traffic accident
Pos.	Positive		RTI	Respiratory tract infection
Post.	Posterior		Rv.	Review
Post Op.	Post operation		RV	Right ventricle
PR	Per rectum		Rx.	Treatment
Prem.	Premature			
Premed.	Premedication		**S**	
Pre Op	Pre operation		s	Second
p.r.n.	As required		SA	Spinal anaesthetic
PTSD	Post traumatic stress disorder		SAD	Seasonal affective disorder
PU	Passed urine		SAH	Sub arachnoid haemorrhage
PUD	Peptic ulcer disease		SaO2	Oxygen saturation
PV	Per vagina		SB	Seen by
			SBR	Serum bilirubin rate
Q			SC	Subcutaneous
q.d.s./q.i.d.	Four times daily		SIDS	Sudden infant death syndrome
Quads.	Quadriceps		SLT	Speech and language therapy/therapist
R			Snr.	Senior
RBC	Red blood cells		SOB	Shortness of breath
RBg	Random blood glucose		SR	Sinus rhythm
RC	Roman Catholic		ST	Sinus tachycardia
RCN	Registered children's nurse		STAT	At once/Immediately
RD	Retinal detachment		Stats.	Statistics
RDS	Respiratory distress syndrome		STM	Short-term memory
Re.	Regarding		Surg.	Surgical
Rec'd	Received			
Recom.	Recommended		**T**	
Reg.	Registrar		TB	Tuberculosis
Rehab.	Rehabilitation		TBL	Total blood loss
REM	Rapid eye movement		TCI	To come in
Reps.	Repetition		T1DM	Type 1 diabetes mellitus
Resp.	Respiration		T2DM	Type 2 diabetes mellitus
Rev.	Revision		t.d.s./t.i.d.	Three times daily
RgN	Registered general nurse		TEDS	Thrombo-embolic deterrent stockings
Rh.	Rhesus		Temp.	Temperature
RICE	Rest, ice, compression, elevation			

TF	Transfer	**W**		
TIA	Transient ischaemic attack	WB	Weight bear/bearing
TPN	Total parenteral nutrition	WBC	Whole blood count
TPR	Temperature, pulse and respiration	WC	Water closet/toilet
		WCC	White cell count
Ts and As	Tonsillectomy and adenoidectomy	W.chair	Wheelchair
		W.end	Weekend
TSH	Thyroid stimulating hormone	WL	Waiting list
		WNL	Within normal limits
U		WR	Ward round
UA	Urinalysis	Wt.	Weight
UC	Urinary catheter		
UANDE	Urea and electrolytes	**X**	
UO	Urinary output	x-match	Crossmatch
URTI	Upper respiratory tract infection	**Y**	
US/USS	Ultrasound/ultrasound scan	YO	Year old
UST	Ultrasound therapy	**Z**	
UTI	Urinary tract infection	Zn	Zinc
V			
Via	By way of	&	And
Vol.	Volume	@	At
VT	Ventricular tachycardia	#	Fracture
VVs	Varicose veins	?	Query
Vx.	Vertex	x2	Twice
		°	Degrees – only permitted for measuring angles
		°C	Temperature in degrees Celsius

(HSE, 2010)

ACTIVITY

Find the full terms for the abbreviations below:

Medical abbreviation	Full term
BD	
PRN	
Hr	
IM	
PO	
ADL	
AandE	
BBA	
BMI	
BNO	
CNS	
DVT	
ENT	
HX	
FH	

References

An Bord Altranais, *Recording Clinical Practice – Guidance to Nurses and Midwives*, Dublin: ABA 2002.

Henderson, B. and Dorsey, J., *Medical Terminology for Dummies*, Indiana: Wiley Publishing 2009, 17–24.

HSE, 'Code of Practice for Healthcare Records Management' available at www.hse.ie/eng/services/Publications/services/Hospitals/NHO_Code_of_Practice_for_Healthcare_Records_Management_Version_2_0.pdf (2010) (accessed 29/7/13).

HSE, *HSE Standards and Recommended Practices for Healthcare Records Management*, QPSD-D-006-3 V3.0, Dublin: HSE 2011, 29, 78.

Infection Prevention and Control

At the end of this chapter the learner should be able to:

- display knowledge of commonly occurring infections, including
  - the organisms that cause them
  - the modes of transmission of these organisms
  - the effects of each infection and how to prevent infection and cross-infection
  - the chain of infection
- demonstrate knowledge of hand hygiene and hand-washing techniques including the five moments for hand hygiene
- demonstrate correct procedure for hand washing and use of alcohol hand rub

Why is infection prevention and control so important?

All healthcare providers have a responsibility to protect their patients, their staff and visitors attending the facility. Good infection-control policies and adherence to the policies demonstrate good and responsible practice. By reducing rates of infection, costs to the healthcare facility are also reduced.

In this chapter we will explore microbiology, different types of infections and the chain of infection. We will also consider hospital-acquired infections, standard precautions and good hand-hygiene practices.

Microbiology

- Microbiology is the branch of science that deals with micro-organisms, or life too small to be seen with the naked eye.

- A microbe is a minute life form – a micro-organism – especially a bacterium that causes disease.

- Microbes are found in all environments but cannot be seen by the naked eye; they measure smaller than 0.1 mm.

- They have many beneficial aspects (food web, nutrient cycling).

- Only a minority is pathogenic and includes germs, viruses, protozoans and bacteria.

- Most of our problems are caused by microbes.

(Wilson, 2006)

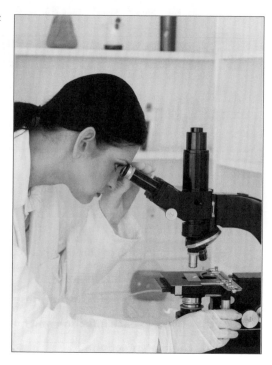

Timeline of microbiology

Microbiology started with the invention of the microscope.

1632–1723: Anton van Leeuwenhoek, a Dutch draper and scientist, became the first man to make and use a real microscope.

1676: He discovered bacteria.

1665: Hooke published the book *Micrographia* which included pictures of objects which he studied through a microscope he built himself.

1796: Edward Jenner was a physician who introduced the smallpox vaccine in 1796.

1822–95: Louis Pasteur studied how yeasts (fungi)

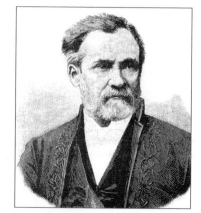

Louis Pasteur

ferment wine and beer, proved that heat destroys bacteria and fungi and found the link between bacteria and infection; the 'germ theory' of disease; pasteurisation.

1818–65: Ignaz Semmelweiss, an obstetrician based in Vienna, studied puerperal ('childbed') fever, a bacterial infection contracted by women during childbirth. He established that high maternal mortality rates were due to the failure of doctors to wash their hands after conducting post-mortems, but was ignored and ridiculed by colleagues.

1857: Joseph Lister, a Scottish surgeon, built on Pasteur's work. He was concerned about infections of compound fractures and post-operative wounds and developed carbolic acid spray to disinfect instruments, patients' and surgeons' skin, thus reducing mortality rates from post-operative wounds.

1843–1910: Robert Koch, a German general practitioner, grew bacteria in culture medium and demonstrated which bacteria caused particular diseases.

1900: Walter Reed, while stationed in Cuba, discovered that yellow fever is transmitted to humans by mosquitoes.

1922: Alexander Fleming discovered penicillin.

(www.theguardians.com/Microbiology)

Bacteria

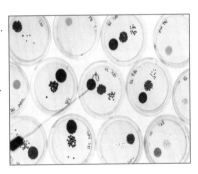

Bacteria are microscopic organisms found everywhere. You cannot see, taste or smell most bacteria. Not all bacteria are harmful (pathogenic); some are beneficial, for example some change milk into cheese. Some people carry bacteria in their nose without suffering ill health; this is known as **colonisation**. However when a bacterium enters a different part of the body, perhaps through a break in the skin, it can multiply and cause illness. This is known as **infection** (HPSC, 2008).

Bacterial organisms grow in a variety of conditions which makes managing them difficult:

- some are O_2 dependent
- some will not grow in O_2
- many love heat (5°C–60°C) and H_2O
- some like dark, others need light

Bacterial infections

There are three classifications of bacterial infection:

1. *Staphylococcus aureus* (*Staph.*)
2. *Streptococcus* (*Strep.*)
3. *Escherichia coli* (*E. coli*)

Staphylococcus aureus (*Staph.*) is a common bacterium. It is found on the skin and in the nose of humans but does not necessarily cause harm. Examples of *Staph. aureus* infection include:

- skin infections (cellulitis and impetigo)

- pneumonia

- food poisoning (*Salmonella, Listeria*)

Mode of transmission

Staph. aureus is spread by direct person-to-person contact (unwashed hands, for example) or by indirect contact; touching something already contaminated with the bacteria (a door handle, for example).

Treatment

Most strains are treated with penicillin-type antibiotics and good hand-hygiene practices. However Methicillin-Resistant *Staphylococcus aureus* (MRSA) is a strain that is resistant to a range of antibiotics. Alternative antibiotics are used on patients with this infection (HPSC, 2008).

Streptococcal infections (*Strep.*)

There are two types: Group A and Group B.

Group A Strep. (GAS) is found on the skin and in the throat. Most carriers have no ill effects from it. The bacterium causes

- *Strep.* throat – a sore, red throat, sometimes with white spots on the tonsils
- scarlet fever – a red rash on the body

Mode of transmission

GAS is spread by skin contact, kissing and sneezing.

Treatment

Prompt antibiotic treatment is recommended.
(HPSC, 2012)

Invasive Strep. A infections

When Strep. A bacteria penetrate into the tissues and organs of the body this is called an invasive infection and requires urgent hospital care and intravenous antibiotic treatment. Examples of invasive infection include:
- pneumonia – an infection of the lungs
- meningitis – an infection of the protective layer that covers the brain

(HSE, 2011)

Group B Strep. (GBS) infection is rare as most people develop natural immunity over their lifetime. However newborn babies are particularly at risk if the mother is *Strep.* B positive. *Strep.* B infections in babies are also rare, affecting only 1 in every 2,000 births.

Mode of transmission

GBS can be transferred from mother to baby in the womb or in the birth canal. However not every colonised mother will pass the bacteria on to her baby.

Treatment

The recommended practice is administration of intravenous antibiotics in labour if the mother is *Strep.* B positive to prevent complications with the baby, in particular pneumonia and meningitis.

Babies considered at risk of developing GBS are commenced on antibiotics following birth.
(HSE, 2011)

Escherichia coli (E. coli)

Escherichia coli (*E. coli*) is a bacterium that normally lives in the intestines. Most types of *E. coli* are harmless, but some can cause sickness and diarrhoea.

Mode of transmission

Contaminated foods are the most common source of infection.

Treatment

Most incidences of *E. coli* resolve without treatment in five to ten days. It is important to maintain good hygiene practices and high standards of food safety (HSE, 2013).

Viral infections

Viruses are very tiny, much smaller than bacteria, and live in our environment all the time just waiting for a host cell to come along. They enter the body through the nose, mouth or breaks in the skin and once inside, they find a host cell to infect. They invade normal healthy cells and use them to multiply, producing more viruses and killing the original healthy cell, causing illness. Examples of viral infections include:

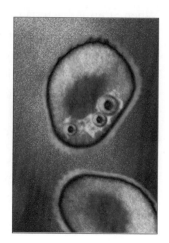

- common cold

- influenza

- warts

- HIV and AIDS

- hepatitis

Mode of transmission

Viruses enter the body via the nose, mouth or breaks in the skin.

Sequence of events leading to a cold

- An infected person sneezes near you.
- You inhale the virus particle, which attaches to cells lining the sinuses in your nose.
- The virus attacks the cells lining the sinuses and rapidly reproduces new viruses.
- The host cells break, and new viruses spread into your bloodstream and also into your lungs. Because you have lost cells lining your sinuses, fluid can flow into your nasal passages and give you a runny nose.
- Viruses in the fluid that drips down your throat attack the cells lining your throat and give you a sore throat.
- Viruses in your bloodstream can attack muscle cells and cause muscle aches.

(Freudenrich, 2012)

Treatment

Antibiotics do not work on viral infections. Vaccines can prevent infection, for example the annual 'flu jab', or the Hepatitis B vaccine for healthcare workers.

Fungal infections

Fungal infections usually affect the skin because they live off keratin, a protein that makes up skin, hair and nails. Examples include:

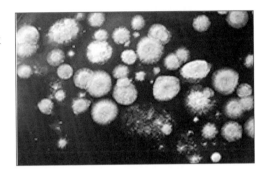

- athlete's foot

- ringworm

- yeast infections

  ‣ intertrigo (in the folds of the skin)

  ‣ thrush

Mode of transmission

- direct contact with another person or an animal that has a fungal skin infection
- indirect contact with contaminated items, e.g. clothes, towels and bedclothes
- walking barefoot in shower and pool areas
- not drying yourself after sweating or bathing
- wearing tight clothing that doesn't allow sweat to evaporate
- cutting or grazing the surface of your skin

Treatment

Treatments are available in the form of creams, lotions, paints, shampoos and medicated powders (HSE, 2012).

Prions

Prions are infectious particles made of mutated protein. They can replicate and cause disease but have no genetic material, which makes prions much tougher than viruses or bacteria. They can survive extremes of heat and radiation and routine theatre sterilisation is insufficient to kill them. Antibiotic and antiviral medicines have no effect on them. Prions kill brain cells and make holes in the brain, causing it to become sponge-like; patients develop Creutzfeldt-Jakob disease (CJD).

There are four types of CJD. Each has a different cause:

- Sporadic CJD (sCJD) is the most common form, accounting for 85 per cent of CJD cases. The cause is unknown. It normally affects people aged over forty.

- Variant CJD (vCJD) was first identified in 1996. vCJD is caused by eating meat from cattle infected with BSE (sometimes called mad cow disease). vCJD mainly affects people in their twenties. Most cases occurred in the UK and vCJD is very rare in Ireland. The number of cases in the UK peaked in 2000 and is now declining.

- Iatrogenic CJD (iCJD) is where the infection is spread from someone with CJD through medical or surgical treatment. Nowadays cases are extremely rare.

- Inherited prion disease (IPD) is a rare form of prion disease caused by inheriting a faulty gene that produces prions.

(HSE, 2012)

Treatment

Unfortunately there is no cure for CJD. The prognosis is poor and most patients die six months to a year following diagnosis (HSE, 2012).

Protozoan infections

Protozoa are single-celled bacteria. They cause infections, the most common of which is malaria (Wilson, 2006). Malaria is a serious tropical disease spread by mosquitoes, which can be fatal if not diagnosed and treated promptly. One bite from a mosquito can cause an infection. Symptoms of malaria include a high temperature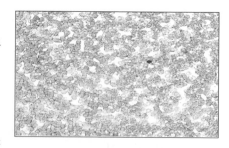
(fever) of 38°C or above, vomiting, sweats and chills, muscle pains, headaches and diarrhoea.

Mode of transmission

Parasites are injected into the body by an infected mosquito.

Treatment

Prompt treatment is vital to recovery. Anti-malarial medication is used both to treat and prevent malaria.

Preventing malaria

If travelling to an area where contracting malaria is a possibility commence anti-malaria medication as prescribed by your GP. Most malaria tablets have to be continued for up to four weeks following your holiday to cover possible incubation (NHS, 2012).

Chain of infection

In order to understand infection prevention and control in more detail we use the 'chain of infection' model. There are six links in the chain, as follows:

Infectious agent

- bacteria
  - ‣ *E. coli*
  - ‣ MRSA
  - ‣ *Streptococcus*
- viruses and prions
  - ‣ influenza
  - ‣ common cold
  - ‣ CJD
- fungi
  - ‣ thrush
  - ‣ athlete's foot
- protozoa
  - ‣ malaria
- worms

Reservoir

- people
  - ‣ normal flora
  - ‣ *Strep.*
  - ‣ *E. coli*
- equipment

> ‣ soil (tetanus)
- water
  > ‣ *Legionella*
- animals and birds
  > ‣ *Salmonella*
  > ‣ *Cryptosporidium*

Portal of exit
- mouth
- nose
- anus
- urethra
- breaks in the skin

Means of transmission
How the infectious agent travels from the portal of exit:
- airborne (TB)
- droplet (common cold, flu)
- contact
  > ‣ indirect (unwashed hands)
  > ‣ direct (sexual contact)
- common vehicle (food, water, blood)
- blood-borne (needle stick, STI)
- vector-borne (mosquitoes)

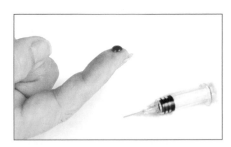

Portal of entry
- inhalation (nose and mouth)
  > ‣ common cold, flu, measles and TB
- ingestion (mouth)
  > ‣ *Salmonella*, cholera, polio
- inoculation (breaks in the skin)
  > ‣ MRSA, malaria and hepatitis B

- urethra/vagina
  - ▸ sexual transmitted infections – gonorrhoea, herpes
- transplacental (during pregnancy)
  - ▸ rubella

Susceptible host

People vulnerable to infection:

- extremes of age
  - ▸ very young and elderly
- drug treatments
  - ▸ chemotherapy
  - ▸ radiation
- underlying medical conditions
  - ▸ diabetes
  - ▸ cystic fibrosis
- anyone with a break in the skin
  - ▸ trauma patients
  - ▸ post-operative patients

We have immunity to some infections from previous exposure and vaccination and babies receive immunity from their mothers in the first three months of life. (Wilson, 2006; HPSC, 2012)

Breaking the chain

How to break the chain of infection, ideally at the early stages:

Infectious agent –prompt identification of the agent of decontamination can greatly reduce risk of transmission.

Reservoir – good hygiene practices, especially disinfection and sterilisation, good employee health and environmental sanitation.

Portal of exit – hand hygiene, appropriate use of personal protective equipment (PPE), good cleaning practices and waste disposal.

Mode of transmission – hand hygiene, airflow control, proper food handling system, sterilisation and disinfection.

Portal of entry – hand hygiene, aseptic technique, wound care, catheter care.

Susceptible host – treat primary illness, recognise potential risk.

FIGURE 8.1: CHAIN OF INFECTION

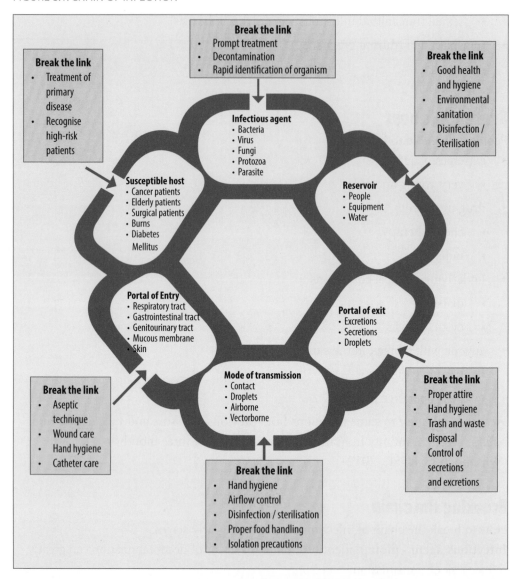

Select an infection and identify each link in the chain of infection relevant to the chosen infection. Describe how the chain of infection might be broken.

Standard precautions

'The purpose of Standard Precautions is to break the chain of infection focusing particularly but not exclusively on the mode of transmission, portal of entry and

susceptible host sections of the chain'
(HPSC, 2009:6).

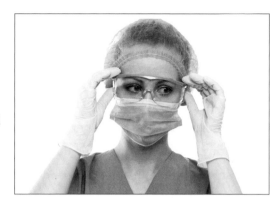

Standard precautions are practices
that should be followed by all
healthcare workers. They work on the
theory that every patient has a potential
infection which could be transmitted.
Practices to manage contact with
body fluids and to minimise risk of
transmission of infection include:

- maintaining hand hygiene

- appropriate use of personal protective equipment (PPE)

  ‣ disposable gloves

  ‣ plastic aprons

  ‣ face masks

  ‣ safety glasses, goggles, visors

  ‣ head protection

  ‣ foot protection

  ‣ fluid repellent gowns

- following unit policy for management of blood and body fluid spillages

- isolating patients or group of patients with the same infection

- adhering to safe use and disposal of sharps

- following needle stick injury policy

- correct disposal of waste and laundry

- ensuring the environment is clean and
  equipment is decontaminated correctly

- following local policies and procedures in
  relation to standard precautions

(HPSC, 2008)

Transmission-based precautions

Transmission-based precautions are contact,
airborne and droplet precautions.

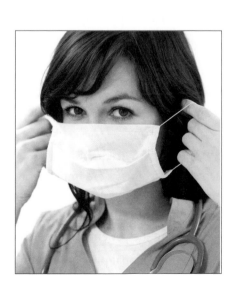

Contact precautions

Contact precautions are implemented in addition to standard precautions to prevent the transmission of highly infectious organisms by direct or indirect contact (MRSA). These extra precautions include

• nursing the patient in isolation in a private room

• wearing gloves for patient contact

• wearing a gown and removing the gown before leaving the room

• washing hands with antiseptic hand wash immediately after leaving the room

• limiting moving the patient

• ensuring equipment, if shared with other patients, is cleaned and disinfected between patients

Always follow local policies and procedures in relation to transmission-based precautions.

Airborne precautions

Airborne precautions are implemented in addition to standard precautions to prevent transmission of highly infectious organisms by air from one person to another (e.g. tuberculosis). These extra precautions include

• nursing the patient in an isolation room

• use of personal protective equipment

  ‣ face mask when caring for patient, put on before entering room and take off after leaving

  ‣ if exposure to respiratory fluids is involved, wear gloves, gown, goggles or face shield

• hand hygiene

• once patient is discharged leave room vacant for one hour and use a mask when cleaning room

Droplet precautions

Droplet precautions are implemented in addition to standard precautions to prevent transmission of highly infectious organisms by respiratory secretions from one person to another (e.g. influenza). These extra precautions include

• nursing the patient in an isolation room

• use of personal protective equipment

  ▸ a face mask for close contact with patient
  ▸ if exposure to 'spray' is involved, gloves, gown and goggles should also be worn
- hand hygiene
- if patient has to leave room make sure they wear a face mask
- clean and disinfect the room on patient discharge

(HPSC, 2008 and CDC, 2011)

Healthcare-associated infections

A healthcare-associated infection, also known as a nosocomial infection, is acquired after contact with the healthcare services. This is most frequently after treatment in a hospital, but can also happen after treatment in outpatient clinics, nursing homes and other healthcare settings. Healthcare-associated infections that are picked up in hospital are also known as hospital-acquired infections (HAI) (HSE, 2013).

The most common type of HAI are

1. surgical wound infection
2. pneumonia
3. urinary tract infection
4. bloodstream infection
5. gastroenteritis

(HSE, 2013)

> ## ACTIVITY
>
> MRSA, *Clostridium difficile* and norovirus are common HAI. Identify the signs and symptoms for each, their mode of transmission and what precautions are necessary when caring for a patient with each infection.

Costs of HAI
- direct cost to HSE for extended hospital stay, extra resources, extra treatment, extra equipment and extra community care for patients who need follow-up care after discharge
- direct cost to patient and family for pain and scarring, extended stay away from family, working days lost, family income loss, financial strain, increased visiting etc., increased morbidity, increased mortality

Hand hygiene

Hand hygiene is recognised as the single most important procedure in preventing hospital acquired infection (HSE, 2013). There are two categories of micro-organisms on the skin: resident flora and transient flora.

- Resident flora
  - ‣ protective function
  - ‣ not easily removed by routine hand washing
  - ‣ can cause infection only when introduced via skin breaks
- Transient flora
  - ‣ acquired through direct contact with another person or object
  - ‣ loosely attached to skin surface and easily transferred by direct contact
  - ‣ easily removed with routine hand hygiene
  - ‣ most abundant around finger tips
  - ‣ important source of cross-infection

Indications for hand washing

- before and after handling invasive devices
- before and after dressing wounds
- before and after contact with immuno-compromised patients
- before and after handling food and drink
- after handling equipment contaminated with body fluid
- after contact with blood or body fluid
- after handling clinical waste and used laundry
- after removing gloves
- after using the toilet
- before leaving the clinical area

(Wilson, 2006:160)

In 2006 the World Health Organization launched the 'five moments for hand hygiene' approach. Each 'moment' defines a key need to perform hand hygiene. They are presented in an easy-to-learn manner which eliminates confusion and conflicting information.

FIGURE 8.2: FIVE MOMENTS FOR HAND HYGIENE

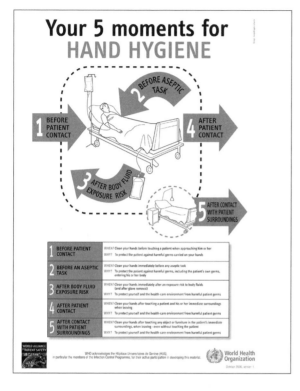

Types of hand washing

Soap and water

Wash your hands with plain soap and water if your hands are visibly soiled (dirty) or contaminated with body fluids, before eating and after using the toilet.

Alcohol hand rub

If your hands are *not* visibly soiled or contaminated with blood or body fluids, use an alcohol-based hand rub routinely to clean your hands before and after direct contact with patients, body fluid or blood, after removing gloves.

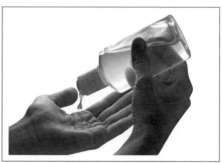

FIGURE 8.3: HAND WASHING – AREAS MISSED

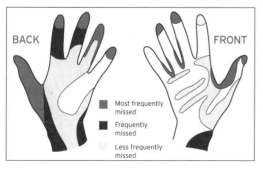

Aqueous antiseptic solutions

Use prior to surgical procedures.

Taylor (1978) identified that 89 per cent of the hand surface is missed when washing, and that the areas of the hands most often missed were the fingertips, finger-webs, palms and the thumbs.

How to wash your hands

- Wet your hands with warm water and apply a small amount of soap on to your hands.
- Rub your hands together until the soap forms lather. Rub all over the top of your hands, in between your fingers and around and under your fingernails.
- Continue to do this for 15 seconds, which is around the length of time it takes to sing the 'Happy Birthday' song twice.
- Rinse your hands well under running water and dry your hands using paper, a clean towel or a hot air dryer.

(HSE, 2013)

FIGURE 8.4: CORRECT SEQUENCE FOR HAND WASHING

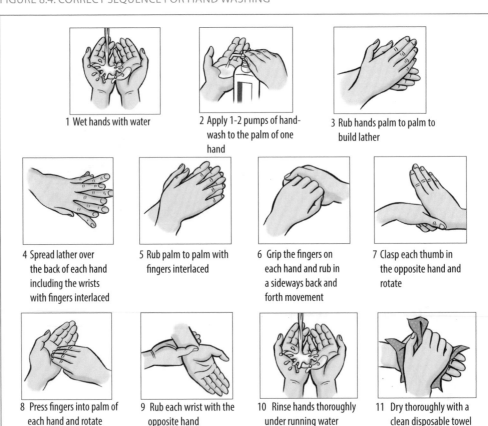

1 Wet hands with water

2 Apply 1-2 pumps of hand-wash to the palm of one hand

3 Rub hands palm to palm to build lather

4 Spread lather over the back of each hand including the wrists with fingers interlaced

5 Rub palm to palm with fingers interlaced

6 Grip the fingers on each hand and rub in a sideways back and forth movement

7 Clasp each thumb in the opposite hand and rotate

8 Press fingers into palm of each hand and rotate

9 Rub each wrist with the opposite hand

10 Rinse hands thoroughly under running water

11 Dry thoroughly with a clean disposable towel

In all healthcare facilities posters demonstrating the correct sequence for hand washing are positioned above wash-hand basins, and posters demonstrating the correct sequence for applying alcohol hand gel are positioned beside dispensers.

FIGURE 8.5: CORRECT SEQUENCE FOR APPLYING ALCOHOL HAND GEL

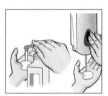

1 Apply gel to the palm of one hand

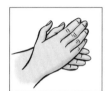

2 Cover whole surface of hands up to wrists, rubbing palm to palm

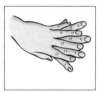

3 Spread gel over the back of each hand including the wrists with fingers interlaced

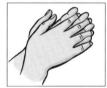

4 Rub palm to palm with fingers interlaced

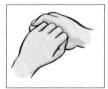

5 Grip the fingers on each hand and rub in a sideways back and forth movement

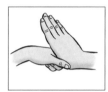

6 Clasp each thumb in the opposite hand and rotate

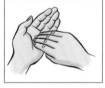

7 Press fingers into palm of each hand and rotate

8 Rub each wrist with the opposite hand

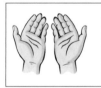

9 Once dry, your hands are safe

ACTIVITY

Practise your hand washing technique with both soap and water and alcohol hand rub. You need to be competent in this skill prior to work placement.

Revision

1.   What conditions do microbes need to grow?
2.   Identify the different types of infections and give two examples of each.
3.   List each link in the chain of infection and give an example for each one.
4.   How can we break the chain of infection?
5.   What is the difference between standard and transmission-based precautions?
6.   What are HAI? Give five examples.
7.   Identify the three types of hand washing and when you should use each type.
8.   Explain the difference between resident and transient flora.
9.   Why is cleaning your hands between patients important?
10. What is PPE? Give five examples of commonly used PPE.

References

Burns, K. *et al.*, HPSC Point Prevalence Survey of Hospital Acquired Infections and Antimicrobial use in European Acute Care Hospitals 2012, Dublin: HPSC 2012.

CDC, 'Basic infection control and prevention plan for outpatient oncology settings' available at www.cdc.gov/HAI/settings/outpatient/basic-infection-control-prevention-plan-2011/transmission-based-precautions.html (2011) (accessed 25/7/13).

Freudenrich, C., 'How viruses work' available at http://science.howstuffworks.com/life/cellular-microscopic/virus-human3.htm (2012) (accessed 23/7/13).

HIQA, 'National Standards for Safer Better Healthcare' available at www.hiqa.ie/standards/health/safer better healthcare (2012) (accessed 24/7/13).

HSE, 'Adult oral thrush' available at www.hse.ie/eng/health/az/O/Oral-thrush-in-adults/ (2012) (accessed 23/7/13).

HSE, 'Athletes foot' available at www.hse.ie/eng/health/az/A/Athlete's-foot/ (2012) (accessed 23/7/13).

HSE, 'Candidiasis, oral (babies)' available at www.hse.ie/eng/health/az/T/Thrush,-oral-babies/ (2012) (accessed 23/7/13).

HSE, 'Fungal nail infection' available at www.hse.ie/portal/eng/health/az/F/Fungal-nail-infection/ (2012) (accessed 23/7/13).

HSE, 'Hand hygiene in Irish healthcare settings' available at www.hse.ie/go/handhygiene (2013) (accessed 25/7/13).

HSE, 'Prions' available at www.hse.ie/portal/eng/health/az/P/Prion-disease/ (2012) (accessed 23/7/13).

HPSC, 'Information leaflet for patients with invasive group A streptococcal infection' available at www.hpsc.ie/hpsc/A-Z/Other/GroupAStreptococcalDiseaseGAS/ Factsheets/FAQforPatients/Title,4535,en.html (2012) (accessed 23/7/13).

HPSC, Standard Precautions Version 1, Dublin: HPSC and HSE 2009, 6.

HPSC, 'Staphylococcus aureus and MRSA' available at www. hpsc.ie/hpsc/A-Z/MicrobiologyAntimicrobialResistance/ EuropeanAntimicrobialResistanceSurveillanceSystemEARSS/ ReferenceandEducationalResourceMaterial/SaureusMRSA/Factsheets/ MainBody,1311,en.html (2008) (accessed 23/7/13).

'Microbiology the beginning: some famous microbiologists and their breakthroughs' available at www.theguardians.com/Microbiology/gm_mbi03.htm (1999) (accessed 23/7/13).

National Institute of Health, 'Bacterial infections' available at www.nlm.nih.gov/ medlineplus/staphylococcalinfections.html (2012) (accessed 23/7/13).

NHS choices, 'Malaria – Introduction' available at www.nhs.uk/Conditions/Malaria/ Pages/Introduction.aspx (2012) (accessed 24/7/13).

SARI, *Guidelines for Hand Hygiene in Irish Health Care Settings*, Dublin: HSE and HPSC 2005.

Taylor, L. J., 'An evaluation of handwashing techniques 2', *Nursing Times* 74(3):108 (1978), 10.

WHO, 'Your 5 moments for hand hygiene' available at www.who.int/gpsc/ tools/5momentsHandHygiene_A3.pdf (2006) (accessed 12/9/13).

Wilson, J., *Infection Control in Clinical Practice*, 3rd ed., Edinburgh: Elsevier 2006, 160.

9

Medication Management

LEARNING OBJECTIVES

At the end of this chapter the learner should be able to:

- explain the importance of precision in administering drugs
- outline what is meant by management and administration of medication
- outline how a nurse/midwife's code of conduct and scope of practice are interlinked with medication administration
- identify the role of the nurse/midwife and the healthcare provider in medication management and administration
- name the 'rights' of medication management
- explain how and why it is important to document drug prescription and administration of medication correctly
- identify key factors which determine the scope of practice for medication management
- explain what Scheduled Controlled/MDA drugs are
- outline key responsibilities for nurses and midwives in relation to monitoring and documenting medication
- explain the importance of educating service users about their medications
- identify correct storage methods for medication
- explain what medication errors and near misses are and outline what a nurse/midwife should do if these occur
- explain why it is important to document and review drugs administration correctly
- identify why it is important to have good numeracy skills in nursing
- outline the entry requirements for registered nurse prescribers in Ireland

Medication management – importance of precision

The nursing, midwifery, medical and pharmaceutical professions are all participants in medication management and contribute to patient/service user care (An Bord Altranais, 2007). While the role of the nurse and midwife in medication administration has changed in recent years, the main responsibility of the nurse's and midwife's role in medication management remains the same and as their *Code of Professional Conduct* (2007) states, 'the nursing profession demands a high standard of professional behaviour from its members and each registered nurse is accountable for his or her practice to deliver and maintain the highest standards of care and safety'.

According to Leufer and Cleary-Holdforth (2011), it is estimated that approximately 10,000 preventable errors and 2,000 preventable deaths occur each year in the Republic of Ireland. 83,847 incidents were reported to the Clinical Indemnity Scheme via Starsweb (national online reporting system) in 2009. Ten per cent of these reported incidents were due to medication errors. Examples of the type and number of reported errors are included in Table 1 below.

TABLE 1: EXAMPLES OF REPORTED MEDICATION ERRORS

Type of medication error	Number of reported events
incorrect doses	1,569
missed medication	1,006
administration of incorrect medication	818
incorrect directions or labelling	562
administration of medication to the incorrect patient	176

(Leufer and Cleary-Holdforth, 2011)

Management and administration of medication

The management and administration of medication involves many different procedures depending on the needs of the individual. The *National Standards for Safer Better Healthcare* (2012) as outlined by the Health Information and Quality Authority (HIQA) refer to the clinically effective, cost effective and safe use of medicines to ensure that service users get the maximum benefit from the medicines they need, while at the same time minimising potential harm.

The five Rs of medication management

The national standards also affirm that medication safety involves ensuring the right service user receives the right medication and is given the right dose, at the right time and by the right route. Along with these, management and providers of all healthcare facilities must have appropriate arrangements in place to ensure the safe and effective use of medicines from the time they are sourced, ordered, stored and prescribed until they are dispensed by pharmacy and administered by nursing staff, who must document appropriately, monitor the effect of the medication on the patient, observe for side effects and errors and report to appropriate personnel, and, when appropriate, ensure the correct disposal of medication.

Maintaining the key factors

Five rights of medication administration

The five rights of medication administration as set out in NMBI guidelines should be applied for each patient/service user encounter:

- right medication
- right patient/service user
- right dosage
- right form
- right time

1. The right medication

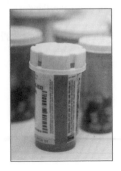

- matching the prescription/medication order against the label of the dispensed medication
- being aware of look-alike and similar-sounding medications
- best practice indicates using generic names of medications whenever possible

2. The right patient/service user

- being certain of the identity of the individual who is receiving the medication
- checking the medical record number and/or identification band
- asking the patient/service user to state her/his name

- confirming that the name and age are a means of ensuring the correct identity

- maintaining a photo of the individual on the medication administration record

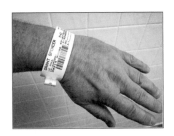

3. The right dosage

- considering if the dosage is appropriate based on age, size, vital signs or other variables

- if it is necessary to measure the dose (e.g. liquid form) ensuring the appropriate equipment is used

- double-checking the dose with a colleague if required by local policy

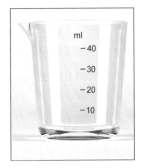

4. The right form (route)

- ensuring that the form, route and administration method of the medication are as prescribed

- if this information is not indicated on the prescription or on the label of the medication, it should be clarified with the prescriber, as many medications can be given by various routes

Medication can be given orally, topically, intravenously, intramuscularly, subcutaneously, per vagina, per rectum or as inhalation.

5. The right time

- ensuring the correct timing, frequency and duration of the prescribed order: this can be vital for ensuring the effectiveness of the drug, e.g. antibiotics: confirm when the last dose was given

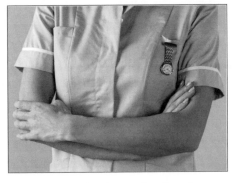

It is important to note that other medication-administration 'rights' have been identified: sometimes eight or nine 'rights' are used.

Elliot and Lui (2010) suggest the following in addition to the five rights listed above.

Right documentation

- Document administration after giving the prescribed medication.

- Chart the time, route, and any other specific information as necessary; for example the site of an injection or any laboratory value or vital sign that needed to be checked before giving the drug.

Right reason

- Confirm the rationale for the ordered medication. What is the patient's history? Why are they taking this medication?

- Revisit the reasons for long-term medication use.

Right response

- Make sure that the drug led to the desired effect. If a diuretic was given, has fluid output increased? Does the patient see an improvement in depression while on an antidepressant?

- Document the monitoring of the patient and any other nursing interventions that are applicable.

- Other vital information includes drug and food interactions and any allergies, health issues, condition, or other contraindications noted due to medication.

It is vital the administrator of the medication has knowledge of medication including generic names, the correct dosage and route as well as the action and side effects of the medication.

Role of the nurse/midwife and health service provider in medication management

An Bord Altranais published *Guidance to Nurses and Midwives on Medication Management* in July 2007, as outlined below.

As part of their role the nurse/midwife should have knowledge of the relevant statutes and legislation regarding the practices of prescribing, dispensing, storing, supplying and administering scheduled medicinal products, including controlled drugs, prescription-only and over-the-counter medication.

Nurses and midwifes have legal and professional accountability with regard to medication management and the health service provider has a responsibility to the service user to assure safe and effective medication management practices.

Scope of practice

The nurse/midwife's professional responsibility regarding medication management is interlinked with their scope of practice (see Chapter 3), which is established and developed from legislation, European directives, international developments, social policy, national and local policies, education and individual levels of competence (An Bord Altranais, 2007).

According to An Bord Altranais (2007), the key factors which determine the scope of practice for medication management are:

- competence
- accountability and autonomy
- continuing professional development
- delegation
- emergency situations

Who administers medication?

Qualified and registered medical and pharmaceutical practitioners, nurses and midwifes may all administer medication.

Medicinal products may normally be administered by a nurse/midwife on their own. As evidenced by best practice, the preparation of a medicinal product should be performed by the same nurse/midwife who administers it to the service user.

According to An Bord Altranais (2007) student nurses/midwives may administer medicinal products under the supervision of a registered nurse/midwife who should follow the principles of supervision. However the registered nurse/midwife retains accountability for the administration of medicinal products.

Double-checking medications

An Bord Altranais (2007) suggests that while registered nurses/midwifes are accountable for their professional decisions and do not need another professional colleague to routinely check their work, and there is no legal or professional requirement that a nurse/midwife must double-check the preparation of a medication with a colleague prior to administration, it can be an important safety check and a means of reducing medication errors. In some areas there are local policies which identify the need to double-check high-alert medications (such as insulin, heparin and chemotherapy) or that require complex calculations in preparation for administration.

Monitoring and documentation of medication management

An Bord Altranais (2007) outlines key responsibilities for nurses and midwives in medication management:

- vital signs and laboratory values prior to administration (as appropriate)
- effectiveness of medication administration method (e.g. is the oral route appropriate for this patient/service user?)
- awareness and observation for medication allergies, possible side effects, adverse reactions, toxicity, interactions and contraindications of medicinal products administered
- monitoring the effectiveness of the administered medicinal products
- the administration of a medicinal product and the patient/service user response should be accurately documented according to local health service policy

The An Bord Altranais (2002) guidelines for good practice in *Recording Clinical Practice* (Section 7) identify that an individual nurse/midwife should establish and maintain accurate, clear and current patient/client records within a legal, ethical and professional framework and the quality of the record-keeping should be such that continuity of care for a patient/client/family is always supported.

While there are many different types of drug chart on which medication prescription and administration are documented, it is vital that the correct details for the service user are on the chart, as well as legible and correct documentation of dosage, name, amount and route of drug as well as signature to confirm that medication has been administered or omitted. Allergies should also be noted.

Response to medication should be recorded in the service user's notes or nursing care plan as per policy and should be reviewed as appropriate.

This attention to detail in medication documentation is necessary to prevent patients receiving wrong medication, over/under-dose of medication, to reduce errors, to report/communicate information to other staff, and to investigate reactions.

If a nurse/midwife is unsure of any detail on the drug chart, they should consult the prescriber of the medication.

MEDICATION CHART

Patient Registration Details	Hospital _____ Prescription Sheet Known Drug Sensitivies/Allergies 1. 2. Patient's Weight

ONCE ONLY AND PRE MEDICATION

Date	Time	Drug	Dose	Route	Signature	Pharm	Time Given	Signature

AS REQUIRED AND POST OPERATIVE DRUGS

Drug Approved Name		Dose	Route	Dose	Time	Date	Signature	Dose	Time	Date	Signature
				1				7			
				2				8			
Frequency	No. of Doses	Date	Pharm	3				9			
				4				10			
Doctor's Signature				5				11			
				6				12			
Drug Approved Name		Dose	Route	Dose	Time	Date	Signature	Dose	Time	Date	Signature
				1				7			
				2				8			
Frequency	No. of Doses	Date	Pharm	3				9			
				4				10			
Doctor's Signature				5				11			
				6				12			
Drug Approved Name		Dose	Route	Dose	Time	Date	Signature	Dose	Time	Date	Signature
				1				7			
				2				8			
Frequency	No. of Doses	Date	Pharm	3				9			
				4				10			
Doctor's Signature				5				11			
				6				12			
Drug Approved Name		Dose	Route	Dose	Time	Date	Signature	Dose	Time	Date	Signature
				1				7			
				2				8			
Frequency	No. of Doses	Date	Pharm	3				9			
				4				10			
Doctor's Signature				5				11			
				6				12			

Patient Registration Details

NB Nursing Staff
CAPITAL letters and APPROVED names are used for drugs
Frequency is specified by ringing time squares
Drug Round times are shown in the front of the binder
Only the following abbreviations may be used: IB, IM and SC

Regular

			Dates → Times ↓												
Drug Approved Name	Dose	Route	0600												
			1000												
Doctor's Signature	Date Written	Date Cancelled	1200												
			1400												
Frequency		Pharm	1800												
			2200												
Drug Approved Name	Dose	Route	0600												
			1000												
Doctor's Signature	Date Written	Date Cancelled	1200												
			1400												
Frequency		Pharm	1800												
			2200												
Drug Approved Name	Dose	Route	0600												
			1000												
Doctor's Signature	Date Written	Date Cancelled	1200												
			1400												
Frequency		Pharm	1800												
			2200												
Drug Approved Name	Dose	Route	0600												
			1000												
Doctor's Signature	Date Written	Date Cancelled	1200												
			1400												
Frequency		Pharm	1800												
			2200												

Patient's Name

FREQUENTLY ADMINISTERED DRUGS OR DRUGS WITH FREQUENT DOSE CHANGES

Doctor's Orders Medication				Medication Given			
Date	Drug	Doctor's Signature	Time	Date	Time	Drug	Nurse's Signature

Patient/service user education

An Bord Altranais (2007) advocates that education should be provided to the patient/service user and/or carer in relation to the use of their medicinal products. It should be explained to the person in a way that is accessible and easy to understand. Consideration should be given to the appropriate timing of teaching, including patient/service user or carer readiness to learn. Best practice would indicate that this information should include:

- the expected mechanism of action of the medicinal product
- potential side effects
- signs and symptoms of potential adverse effects and actions to take if they occur
- possible interactions of the medicinal product with other medications, particular foods or other substances
- precautions or instructions to follow, including time, route, method of administration and storage of medicinal products
- significance of adherence to prescribed therapy (duration and frequency)
- recommendations for follow-up and reporting of potential side effects or adverse reactions

Considerations for withholding medication

At times it is appropriate to exercise professional judgement to withhold a medicinal product if relevant in a specific patient/service user case. An Bord Altranais (2007) states that the medical practitioner or registered nurse prescriber should be contacted with details if contraindications of administration exist, thereby communicating changes in the condition of the patient/service user.

Accurate and contemporaneous documentation should be made for any medicinal product withheld or refused. Any information or advice given to a patient/service user about the possible consequences of such an action should also be documented.

Refusal of medication by a service user

The decision by a patient/service user or parent/guardian to refuse administration of a medicinal product (after having been provided with information about the drug and the risks and benefits of the therapy) should be respected and the medical practitioner or registered nurse prescriber should be notified (An Bord Altranais, 2007).

Emergency situations and the use of verbal and telephone orders

An Bord Altranais (2007) reports that the only acceptable time a verbal or telephone order for medication should be taken from a medical practitioner is in an emergency situation, where there is an immediate unplanned patient/service user need. A nurse or midwife accepting a verbal or telephone order should repeat the order to the medical practitioner for verification.

A record of the verbal or telephone order should be documented in the appropriate section of the patient/service user's medical chart/notes. This should include the date and time of the receipt of the order, the prescriber's full name and their confirmation of the order.

Best practice indicates that, where possible, the medical practitioner should repeat the order to a second nurse or midwife. This should be followed by the nurses/midwives confirming the order between them. The justification and rationale for accepting a verbal or telephone medication order should also be documented by the nurse/midwife involved to establish the clinical judgement exercised in the emergency situation.

The medical practitioner is responsible for documenting the written order on the prescription sheet or medication administration record within an acceptable timeframe as determined by the health service provider. This responsibility also applies in the case of electronic record keeping.

Scheduled controlled/MDA drugs

The Misuse of Drugs Acts, 1977 and 1984 and the Misuse of Drugs Regulations, 1988, 1993 and 2007 determine the conditions of production, possession, supply, importation and exportation of controlled drugs. The drugs are categorised into five schedules with different controls applicable to each category. The legal term for these drugs is the abbreviation MDA accompanied by the appropriate schedule of the drug. For example, MDA Schedule 2 replaces the previous term of CD2.

TABLE 2: EXAMPLES OF SCHEDULES, DRUGS AND CONTROLS IN THE MDA SCHEDULES

Schedule 1	Cannabis, coca leaf, raw opium and hallucinogenic drugs such as LSD	Special licence is required regarding any activity with these drugs

Schedule 2	Opiates (morphine and heroin) amphetamines and synthetic narcotics (pethidine) methadone, hydrocodone	Licence is required for import and export. A pharmacist can only supply to a named individual by special prescription. Safe custody must be maintained. Records of drug activity must be maintained. Records of destruction must be witnessed.
Schedule 3	Barbiturates, potent analgesia, minor stimulants and two benzodiazepines (flunitrazepam and temazepam)	Safe custody of these drugs must be maintained. Special controlled drug prescription.
Schedule 4	Most other benzodiazepines (other than two above)	Control of these drugs is minimal, normal prescription and administration rules of medication apply.
Schedule 5	Preparations (not injection) containing codeine or nicocodeine; preparations of cocaine containing not more than 0.1% calculated as cocaine base	This schedule identifies products exempt from most restrictions under the regulation. Invoices regarding these products must be kept for two years.

(An Bord Altranais, *Guidance to Nurses and Midwives on Medication Management* 2007, Appendix C)

The nurse/midwife manager (or acting manager) in charge of a ward, theatre or department may be supplied with a controlled drug solely for the purpose of administration to patients/service users in that ward, theatre or department, on foot of a requisition issued by them in accordance with the directions of a medical practitioner.

The Misuse of Drugs Regulations, 1988 Article 8 (1)(a) does not pertain to private hospitals and private nursing homes and therefore they have no authority to be in possession of controlled drugs or to be supplied with such drugs. Supplies of controlled drugs for patients/service users in private hospitals and private nursing homes should be obtained by way of a medical prescription as if the patients/service users were in their own homes. Private hospital and private nursing home patients/service users are considered to be in the same position as a patient/service user in their own home (An Bord Altranais, 2007).

Management of MDA Schedule 2 drugs

The local health service provider policy may require two persons to conduct the administration of MDA Schedule 2 drugs, one of whom is a nurse/midwife. This is not a legal requirement. It is recommended that local health service providers should consider including requirements expected for the checking, preparation, administration or destruction of these drugs when establishing medication management policies. They should also consider whether these activities are to be witnessed and by whom (e.g. another nurse/midwife or other member of the healthcare team).

Access to the keys of the controlled drugs storage should be the subject of local policy, bearing in mind responsibility and accountability issues. The nurse/midwife manager or their nurse/midwife designee should keep the keys of the controlled drugs storage on their person.

Policies and procedures should be in place for monitoring/checking a stock balance at each transaction of MDA Schedule 2 drugs. At changeover of shifts, a nurse/midwife from each shift should complete the count of these scheduled drugs.

Appropriate documentation of the administration of MDA Schedule 2 drugs should be entered in the patient/service user's chart/notes and in the ward controlled drugs register.

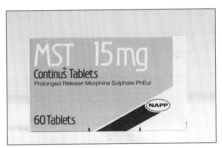

The nurse/midwife manager should keep requisition copies (or a note) detailing the requested MDA Schedule 2 drugs submitted to the pharmacist or nursing/midwifery director who supplies the drugs (An Bord Altranais, 2007) .

Community care involving MDA Schedule 2 drugs

An MDA Schedule 2 drug may be obtained on prescription and retained in the patient/service user's home. In the community, individually prescribed medicinal products, including controlled scheduled drugs, are the property and responsibility of the individual patient/service user.

Where the patient/service user resides in the community

- Nurses/midwives are authorised to transport the drug to a person for whom the drug has been properly prescribed and dispensed by a pharmacist .
- They are not otherwise permitted to have the drug in their possession or storage.

Where the patient/service user is being transported into the community

- The drugs must be dispensed by the pharmacist to the patient/service user on an individual basis as per the written prescription.

- The drugs should not be supplied from the stock of MDA drugs on the ward.

- The Misuse of Drugs Regulations, 1988 allows for the supply of MDA scheduled drugs to patients/service users while in the hospital/nursing home setting but not once they leave and enter the community. These drugs should be stored securely for transport.

- Unused or expired controlled drugs should be returned for destruction to the pharmacy from which they were dispensed (An Bord Altranais, 2007).

Community midwifery and MDA Schedule 2 drugs

- A community midwife is authorised as per the exemptions to the Misuse of Drugs (Amendment) Regulations, 2007 to have in their possession pethidine for their practice.

- A written order is signed by the midwife and countersigned by a medical practitioner or registered nurse prescriber practising in their area.

The medication order must state:

- the name and address of the midwife

- the quantity to be supplied

- the purpose for which it is required

A record must be kept in a book by the midwife of any supply of pethidine that they obtain and administer. The record must include:

- the name and address of the person from whom the drug was obtained

- the amount obtained

- the form in which it was obtained

After administering the pethidine to the patient/service user, the midwife must enter into the book:

- the name and address of the patient/service user

- the amount administered

- the form in which it was administered

This book should be kept for a period of two years from the date on which the last entry was made (An Bord Altranais, 2007).

Storage of medicinal products

An Bord Altranais (2007) outlines that all medicinal products should be stored in a secure manner, either in a locked cupboard or room. They should be stored in the appropriate environment as indicated on the label or packaging of the medicinal product or as advised by the pharmacist.

Controlled or MDA scheduled controlled drugs should be locked in a separate cupboard/container from other medicinal products to ensure further security; usually in a locked cupboard within a locked cupboard.

Medicinal products requiring refrigeration, according to package labelling or the pharmacist, should be stored in a designated refrigerator that is:

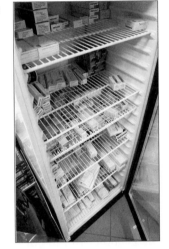

- not used for any other purpose

- accessible and reliable

- capable of being secured

Medicinal products should be stored separately from antiseptics, disinfectants and other cleaning products. Mobile trolleys and emergency boxes storing medicinal products should be locked and secure when not in use.

Policies and procedures should be in place for

- ordering medicinal products from the pharmacy

- checking delivery and inventory of medicinal products to the ward/unit and maintaining records

- the immediate reporting and investigation of discrepancies in medicinal products stocks

- the storage of medicinal products for self-administration by patients/service users

Safety in medication management

Standard precautions and aseptic techniques must be adhered to during all aspects of the preparation and administration of medications. It is also vital that appropriate hand hygiene as per the World Health Organization (WHO) 'Five moments of hand hygiene' and aseptic techniques are used at all times to reduce the risk of cross contamination.

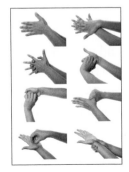

Correct disposal of equipment in a sharps container is vital to prevent the transfer of infection and reduce the risk of a needle-stick injury.

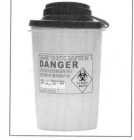

Medication errors and near misses

Medication error is the most common type of error affecting patient/service user safety and is the most common single preventable cause of adverse events (National Medicines Information Centre, 2001). According to Leufer and Cleary-Holdforth (2011), it is necessary to identify and adopt safety measures and where necessary facilitate a culture that will improve patient safety, assist and support nursing professionals and value the people who report errors and near misses.

An Bord Altranais (2007) defines medication errors as preventable events that may cause or lead to inappropriate medication use or patient/service user harm while the medication is in the control of the healthcare professional or patient/service user.

These events may be associated with professional practice, healthcare products, procedures and systems. They include prescribing, order communication, product labelling, packaging and nomenclature, compounding, dispensing, distribution, administration, education, monitoring and use (National Coordinating Council for Medication Error Reporting and Prevention, 1998 cited in An Bord Altranais, 2007). Medication errors can occur at any point in the medication management cycle.

The *Code of Conduct* (2000) states that any circumstance which could place patients/clients in jeopardy or which militates against safe standards of practice should be made known to appropriate persons or authorities.

It is of primary importance upon noting a medication error that the patient/service user's health is monitored. If a medication error has been identified, medical and nursing interventions should be implemented immediately to limit potential adverse effects or reactions. Patient/service user safety is paramount.

Medication errors and near-miss events should be seen as opportunities to assess practice(s), identify what went wrong, learn from mistakes and institute changes to the medication system. The prevention, detection and reduction of medication errors and near misses should be effected with collaboration throughout the healthcare team, as errors may reflect a problem with the system and may involve other professions and departments. It is not the sole responsibility of the prescriber to report adverse reactions to drugs. The members of the healthcare team responsible for monitoring patients also have a role in reporting these cases (An Bord Altranais, 2007).

Continuous quality improvement programmes for monitoring medication errors and near misses should be in place within risk management systems of the organisation. Fostering cultures of safety and continuing professional development in medication management for nurses and midwives is important in preventing and addressing the causes of medication errors.

Numeracy skills in nursing

Warburton (2010) highlights the fact that the ability to perform calculations competently is a basic requirement for all nurses. It is essential for patient safety that nurses are able to competently perform numerical and drug calculations (McMullen, 2010).

Calculations are used in everyday tasks such as working out drug doses, body-mass index and fluid-balance charts. An error due to incorrect calculations can lead to further illness, debilitation or even death. Ongoing education is important for nurses to maintain numeracy skills and all nurses must be aware of the consequences of drug errors due to miscalculation.

Crushing medications

An Bord Altranais (2007) states that nurses or midwives who administer medicines to their patients/service users in a modified form to that prescribed (e.g. crushing an oral medication that is in a tablet or pill form), should ensure that other methods have been considered and that appropriate advice is sought.

The Irish Medicines Board (IMB) is the regulatory body responsible for the licensing or authorisation of medicinal products for human and veterinary use. The IMB states that if a medicinal product is used outside of the instructions as provided for in the posology section of the *Summary of Product Characteristics*, then it is used outside its licensed conditions. This would apply to medications which are crushed.

Only medical and dental practitioners can legally authorise the administration of 'unlicensed' medicines to humans. Consequently, if a nurse or midwife decides that a change in the form of the drug is necessary for its safe administration, they should consult the medical practitioner and pharmacist to discuss alternative preparations or forms of administration for the patient/service user (An Bord Altranais).

If it is deemed necessary to administer the medication in a crushed format, this should be prescribed by the medical practitioner in the patient/service user's medication chart/prescription sheet with the consent of the patient/service user or carer if applicable. Development of a policy to support the practice of crushing oral medications, inclusive of guidelines and decision-making rationale for individual events, should also be considered (An Bord Altranais, 2007).

Adverse drug reactions

According to An Bord Altranais (2007) nurses and midwives are in a prime position to observe and report on suspected adverse reactions. The reporting and monitoring of adverse reactions has significant implications for patient/service user safety. It is not necessary to determine a causal relationship between a drug and subsequent event prior to reporting suspected adverse reactions. Nursing/midwifery staff should liaise with the prescriber about the submission of the report as appropriate. The health service provider's medication management policies should include information and direction for healthcare professionals in reporting suspected adverse reactions.

The Irish Medical Board requests that healthcare professionals (defined as medically qualified persons: nurses, midwives, doctors, dentists, and pharmacists) report the following:

- all suspected reactions to new products
- serious suspected reactions to established products (that is, those available on the market for more than two years)
- any suspected increase in the frequency of minor reactions
- all suspected reactions to vaccines
- all suspected teratogenic (affecting development of foetus) effects

Nurse prescribers in Ireland

In 2001 An Bord Altranais and the National Council for the Professional Development of Nursing and Midwifery conducted a project named Review of Nurses and Midwives in the Prescribing and Administration of Medicinal Products. The final report of this project, published in 2005, provided a number of key recommendations to support the expansion of practice of nurse and midwife prescribing.

In early 2006 the Irish Medicines Board (Miscellaneous Provisions) Act was introduced which contained an enabling provision for prescriptive authority for nurses and midwives. The Minister for Health and Children, in May 2007, signed into law the medicines regulations providing the regulatory framework for this national initiative.

Prescribing is an expansion of a nurse/midwife's scope of practice, beyond the skills, competence and knowledge an individual practitioner possesses at the point of registration.

The professional regulatory framework for nurse/midwife prescribing is established through the *Practice Standards and Guidelines for Nurses and Midwives with Prescriptive Authority* 2010, which set out the professional responsibilities of the nurse and midwife and are viewed as rules within which a nurse/midwife is expected to practise.

DECISION-MAKING FRAMEWORK

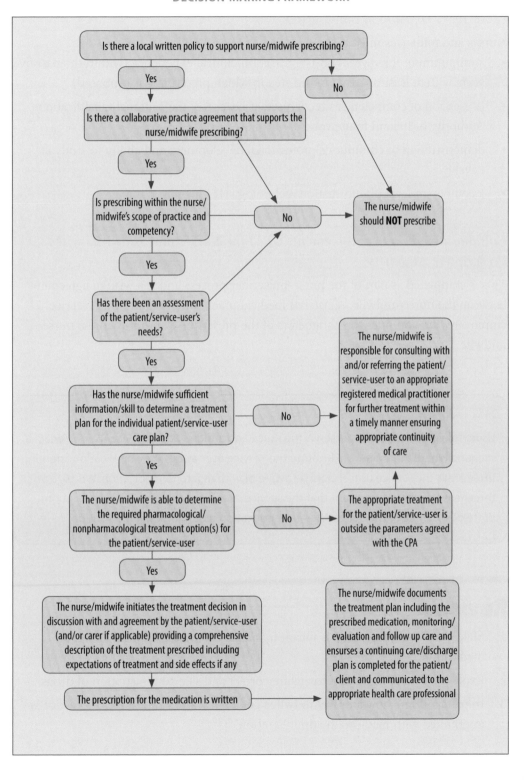

Is there a local written policy to support nurse/midwife prescribing?

Yes

No

Is there a collaborative practice agreement that supports the nurse/midwife prescribing?

Yes

Is prescribing within the nurse/midwife's scope of practice and competency?

No

The nurse/midwife should **NOT** prescribe

Yes

Has there been an assessment of the patient/service-user's needs?

Yes

Has the nurse/midwife sufficient information/skill to determine a treatment plan for the individual patient/service-user care plan?

No

The nurse/midwife is responsible for consulting with and/or referring the patient/service-user to an appropriate registered medical practitioner for further treatment within a timely manner ensuring appropriate continuity of care

Yes

The nurse/midwife is able to determine the required pharmacological/nonpharmacological treatment option(s) for the patient/service-user

No

The appropriate treatment for the patient/service-user is outside the parameters agreed with the CPA

Yes

The nurse/midwife initiates the treatment decision in discussion with and agreement by the patient/service-user (and/or carer if applicable) providing a comprehensive description of the treatment prescribed including expectations of treatment and side effects if any

The nurse/midwife documents the treatment plan including the prescribed medication, monitoring/evaluation and follow up care and ensurses a continuing care/discharge plan is completed for the patient/client and communicated to the appropriate health care professional

The prescription for the medication is written

Minimum entry requirements for admission to registration in the Nurse Prescribers Division of the Register

Nurses and midwives must have

- a minimum of three years post-registration clinical experience (within the past five years with at least one year in the area in which prescribing is proposed)
- possession of competencies recognised at Level 8 of the National Qualifications Authority of Ireland framework
- demonstration of continuous professional development and ability to study at Level 8
- a competent level of information technology (IT) literacy

Collaborative Practice Agreement (CPA) for Nurses and Midwives with Prescriptive Authority

This is completed as part of the nurse-prescriber process and is a written agreement between the nurse/midwife, registered medical practitioner(s) and health service employer which outlines the parameters of the prescriptive authority of the nurse/midwife.

ACTIVITY

Using role play where one person is the nurse and another is the service user, re-enact a scenario where the 'nurse' is educating the 'service user' about their medication. Identify three areas the service user should be aware of with regard to medication. Write down three reasons why it important that the service user is educated on their medications. Write down three barriers to service-user education regarding their medication.

Revision

1. Make notes outlining what is meant by management and administration of medication.
2. Explain why it is important to ensure correct and safe administration of drugs.
3. In pairs, outline how a nurse/midwife's code of conduct and scope of practice is interlinked with medication administration.

4. Discuss the role of the nurse and the healthcare provider in medication management and administration.

5. Using a mind map, illustrate the rights of medication management.

6. According to An Bord Altranais (2007), what are the key factors which determine the scope of practice for medication management?

7. Explain what Scheduled Controlled/MDA drugs are.

8. Outline key responsibilities for nurses and midwives in monitoring and documenting medication.

9. Explain why it is important to document and review drugs administration correctly.

10. Explain what medication errors and near misses are and what a nurse should do if these occur.

11. Identify why it is important to have good numeracy skills in nursing.

12. Outline the requirements that need to be fulfilled prior to becoming a nurse prescriber in Ireland.

References

An Bord Altranais, *Code of Professional Conduct for each Nurse and Midwife*, Dublin: An Bord Altranais 2000.

An Bord Altranais, *Guidelines for Good Practice in Recording Clinical Practice*, Dublin: An Bord Altranais 2002.

An Bord Altranais, *Guidance to Nurses and Midwives on Medication Management*, Dublin: An Bord Altranais 2007.

An Bord Altranais, *Practice Standards for Nurses and Midwives with Prescriptive Authority*, Dublin: An Bord Altranais 2007.

An Bord Altranais, *Scope of Nursing and Midwifery Practice Framework*, Dublin: An Bord Altranais 2000.

Elliot, M. and Lui, Y., 'The nine rights of medication administration: an overview', *British Journal of Nursing* 19:5 (2010), 300–305.

Health Information and Quality Authority, *National Standards for Safer Better Healthcare*, Dublin: HIQA 2012.

Leufer, T. and Cleary-Holdforth, J., 'Medication management: last line of defence' available at www.inmo.ie/tempDocs/MedManagement48-50.pdf (2011).

McMullen, M., 'Exploring the numeracy skills of nurses and students when performing drug calculations' available at www.nursingtimes.net/nursing-practice/clinical-zones/prescribing/exploring-the-numeracy-skills-of-nurses-and-students-when-performing-drug-calculations/5018767.article (2010).

National Medicines Information Centre, *Bulletin on Medication Errors*, Dublin: NMIC 2001.

Warburton, P., 'Numeracy and patient safety: the need for regular staff assessment', *Nursing Standard* 24:27 (2010), 42–4.

10

Safe Moving and Handling Practice

LEARNING OBJECTIVES

At the end of this chapter the learner should be able to:

- identify what is meant by safe handling practice
- explain why it is necessary to learn, develop and practise safe handling techniques
- identify the consequences of poor moving and handling practice
- outline what safe handling training and practice entails
- name the legislation related to manual handling
- name the main components in risk assessment
- list eight principles of safer moving and handling
- list four pieces of equipment used to assist with moving and handling

Safe moving and handling practice

As a part of any course which trains people to work in the care area, it is necessary for the learner to develop knowledge on safe practice and to experience practice in safe handling and moving techniques. The learner usually has the opportunity to obtain up to date certification in Patient Moving and Handling. This chapter provides an introduction to the theory and practice of safe handling and moving and outlines the main components of an appropriate training course.

Background to manual handling and safe lifting practice

Safe moving and handling practice is an essential part of the working life of many people, particularly if they need to move or handle any animate object (for example a person) or inanimate object (for example a box). It is also a life skill, as moving and handling is a part of everyday activities for most people. It is also a legal requirement that employers and employees take responsibility for maintaining safe practice and taking reasonable care of their own and other people's safety.

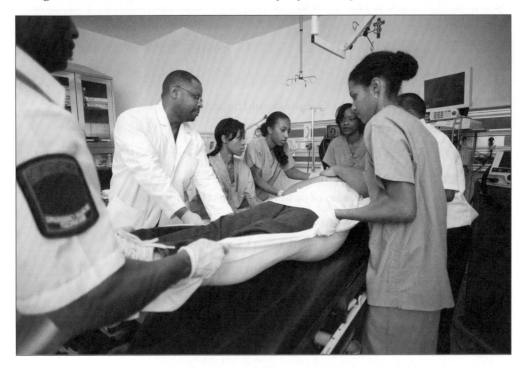

The terms 'manual handling' and 'moving and handling' are used in law and training and to explain and outline the main components of safe practice when lifting, lowering, filling, emptying, carrying or moving animate or inanimate loads. The terms also refer to climbing, pushing, pulling or turning any loads (Health and Safety Authority).

Why is manual handling training necessary?

According to the Health and Safety Authority (HSA), manual handling accounts for thirty-three per cent of accidents reported to their organisation. In the health and social care area the proportion of incidents associated with manual handling is particularly high, reported to be about thirty-eight per cent. Attendants accounted for the highest number of claimants (Dockrell *et al.*, 2007). Nurses are reported to have a high level of back problems associated with manual handling (Waters *et al.*, 2006, Swain *et al.*, 2003).

Consequences of poor moving and handling practice

Dockrell *et al.* (2007), in a report on moving and handling in the healthcare area submitted to the HSA, found that the most common type of injury resulted in physical stress or strain to the body and the most frequently injured body part was the back. The specific details of incidents which caused the most injury as reported by Dockrell *et al.* are outlined in the table below.

Cause of injury	Numbers affected
lifting heavy/awkward load	63.3%; n=22 (includes patients)
handling a falling patient	23.3%; n=8
other	13.3%; n=5

People can get injured as a result of one incident or from repetitive actions. Tasks which lead to injury may involve twisting and bending, repetitive motions, carrying or lifting heavy loads, and standing in fixed positions for a prolonged period.

Poor moving and handling practice can lead to

- back pain and musculo-skeletal disorders, which can lead to inability to work
- moving and handling accidents – which can injure the person being moved, the employee and any other individual involved in the move or lift
- discomfort, fear and a lack of dignity for the person being moved

Education and training

Education and training is a legislative requirement and is a fundamental part of understanding safe handling and moving and preventing injury. It should contain academic, practical and assessment components.

Ongoing practice

Developing safe practice techniques is an ongoing process and requires practice as well as knowledge. Traditionally in Ireland training in manual handling has been considered vital for work practice. However it has been reported that training interventions based primarily on technique training have little impact on work practices or injury rates and knowledge learned in training may not always be applied in practice (Hignett *et al.,* 2003, Swain *et al.*, 2003). Therefore manual handling and moving-and-handling training should be multifaceted and provide learners with the knowledge and skills to carry out a manual handling activity in a manner which reduces or eliminates the risk of injury. The tools developed during training must then be applied in the workplace.

Training courses

It was determined in 2010 that all instructors in manual handling should attain a FETAC Level 6 Manual Handling Instructor qualification or FETAC Level 6 People Handling Instructor qualification (O'Halloran, 2010).

Most training courses for non-care staff should be half-day courses focusing on moving inanimate objects, while individuals who assist people to move tend to complete full-day courses. It is important to remember that patient moving and handling can be more difficult than moving an inanimate object as patients can be unpredictable; they vary in size, mobility, cognitive ability, level of need, condition and the requirement for appropriate resources.

Contents of a manual handling training course

In 2010 the Health and Safety Authority recommended the aims of a manual handling training programme, which are summarised below.

1. **Learners will be aware of the legislative requirements in relation to manual handling.**

    Legalisation which is relevant in manual handling includes the following:

    *   **The Manual Handling of Loads Regulation Part VI of the Safety, Health and Welfare at Work (General Application) Regulations 1993** brought in to Irish legislation the EU Council Directive 90/269/EEC on the minimum health

and safety requirements for the manual handling of loads. Since then there have been additions and new regulations for both employers and employees.

- **The Safety, Health and Welfare at Work (General Application) Regulations 2007** outline the requirements that must be adhered to in relation to manual handling. These regulations are implemented under the Safety, Health and Welfare at Work Act 2005, and contain four key requirements:
  - ‣ avoidance of manual handling
  - ‣ reduction of manual handling
  - ‣ risk assessment of manual handling tasks
  - ‣ provision of instruction and training for relevant employees

2. **Learners will acquire the basic knowledge on risk factors for back problems and in maintaining a healthy back.**

   Our musculo-skeletal system is designed to be able to move objects, but poor posture, incorrect movements and poor ergonomics or workplace conditions can damage it. In order to handle an object safely it is essential to have a knowledge of this system and its flexibility.

3. **Learners will be aware of how to carry out a basic personal/dynamic manual handling risk assessment to determine if the load can be handled safely.**

   Risk assessment is a process which involves gaining a detailed understanding of a task to be carried out, collecting all relevant technical details of the task, identifying if there are risk factors/hazards present, exploring what options or solutions are available to reduce or eliminate the risk factors/hazards and putting a plan in place to introduce the agreed control measures.

   - Learners need to be aware of the specific manual handling hazards in their work area as identified in the task-specific manual handling risk assessment. They should also be familiar with measures to avoid or reduce the risk of injury, including the use of mechanical aids or reorganisation of the work activity.

The Health and Safety Authority has published guidelines to assist with the identification of problems and risks and recommends that risk assessment is carried out as summarised in the table below:

Summary of risk assessment process	
Step 1	Identify the manual handling tasks that need to be assessed
Step 2	Develop a risk assessment schedule
Step 3	Carry out the risk assessment process

Step 3a	Observe and describe task
	(Gain a detailed understanding of how the task is performed)
Step 3b	Collect task data
	(A well-documented manual handling risk assessment will have good quality information about the task)
Step 3c	Identify the risk factors
	(Schedule 3 details the risk factors for the manual handling of loads. This schedule should be consulted in order to identify risk factors in the task)
Step 3d	Develop a solution and action plan
	(This is the process of eliminating or reducing risk factors)
Step 4:	Review the effectiveness of the control measures or solution

Source: *Health and Safety Authority Guide to the Safety, Health and Welfare at Work (General Application) Regulations 2007*

4. Learners will be able to state the main principles of safer manual handling

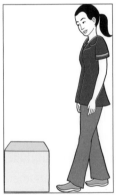

Assess task, area, load

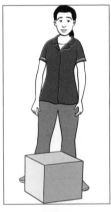

Broad stable base (feet flat on floor)

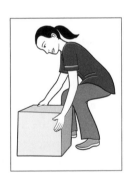

Bend the knees

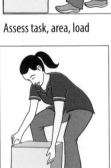

Back straight (not necessarily vertical)

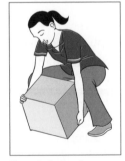

Firm grip (palmer)

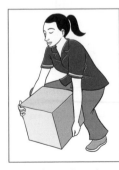

Arms in line with trunk

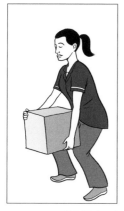 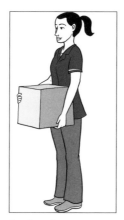 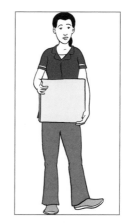 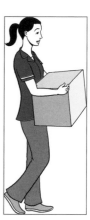

Weight close to centre of gravity   Point feet in the direction of movement

5. **Learners will be able to carry out relevant manual handling techniques and understand the need to further develop these skills in the workplace.**

   • The learner should practise moves and lifts and develop an understanding of how these techniques can be used in the workplace. The learner then needs to continue to use the techniques in the workplace; however they should not take on unsupervised tasks related to manual handling until they are competent to do so.

   • If learners are involved in patient/client handling a training programme should also include the following learning outcomes. The learner

      ‣ needs to be aware of local policies and procedures related to handling patients which are relevant to their work area (such as bariatric guidelines, falls strategies, infection control, hoist management etc.)

      ‣ must be able to identify the additional factors which need to be included in a manual handling risk assessment when handling people; taking into account patient's size, mobility, cognitive ability, condition, needs and resources

      ‣ be aware of written documentation in relation to patient handling risk assessments in their work area and the need to record information related to falls and manual handling issues

      ‣ be aware of a range of handling aids available in their work area and their safe use

      ‣ practise moving and lifting using equipment such as slide sheets and hoists and develop an understanding of how these can be used in the workplace.

The learner then needs to continue to practise in the workplace but should not take on unsupervised tasks related to manual handling until they are competent to do so

▸ participate in a range of core patient handling techniques relevant to their work tasks

It is vital that a risk assessment of any task which involves manual handling is carried out before an informed decision can be made on how to carry out the task.

Moving and handling equipment

The type and amount of equipment needed will vary according to the specific needs of care service users. When providing equipment, employers should consider:

• the needs of the individual – helping to maintain, wherever possible, independence

• the safety of the individual and of staff

Equipment for manual handling should only be used by practitioners who are competent to use it, having received training and assessment and ensuring that equipment is used in accordance with the patient/client's individual needs and manufacturer's instructions.

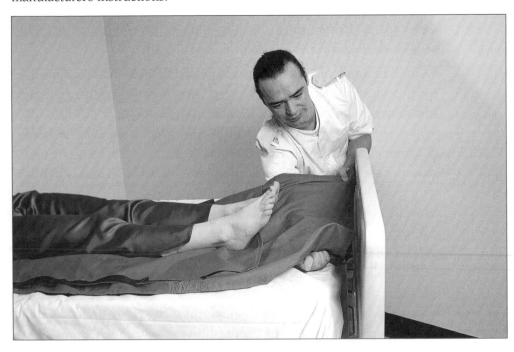

Common manual handling equipment may include

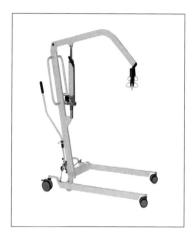

- a variety of hoists – e.g. hoists to raise fallen individuals from the floor, standing hoists, mobile hoists etc.
- slings of different types and sizes
- transfer boards
- bath hoists or bath lifts and/or adjustable height baths
- slide sheets
- turntables
- electric beds – for dependent/immobile residents
- wheelchairs
- handling belts to assist weight-bearing residents (not for lifting)
- bed levers, support rails/poles
- suitable walking aids, hand rails etc. for people needing minor assistance
- bariatric equipment (for use with very heavy people)

Revision

1. What is meant by safe handling practice?
2. Discuss why it is necessary to learn, develop and practise safe handling techniques.
3. Write a note explaining the consequences of poor moving and handling practice.
4. Outline what safe handling training and practice entails.
5. Name the legislation which sets out requirements related to manual handling.
6. Define risk assessment in relation to manual handling.
7. In a simple table format, identify the four main stages used in risk assessment.
8. Using a mind map, name the eight principles of safer manual handling.
9. List four pieces of equipment used to assist with moving and handling.

References

Dockrell, S. *et al.*, 'Report submitted to the Health and Safety Authority' available at www.hsa.ie/eng/Workplace_Health/Manual_Handling/Manual_Handling_Research_Reports/Manual_Handling_Analysis_Report.pdf (2007)

Health and Safety Authority, 'Guide to the Safety, Health and Welfare at Work (General Application) Regulations' available at www.hsa.ie/eng/Publications_and_Forms/Publications/Retail/Gen_Apps_Manual_Handling.pdf (2007) (accessed 26/07/13)

HAS, 'Guidance on the Manual Handling Training System – 2010 Revision' available at www.hsa.ie/eng/Publications__andForms/Publications/Occupational_Health/Manual%20Revision%202.pdf (2010) (accessed 25/07/13)

Hignett, S. *et al.*, *Evidence-Based Patient Handling: Tasks, equipment and interventions*, London: Routledge 2003.

O'Halloran, M., 'Guidance on the Manual Handling Training System – 2010 Revision' available at www.hsa.ie/eng/Publications__andForms/Publications/Occupational_Health/Manual%20Revision%202.pdf (2010) (accessed 25/07/13)

Swain, J. *et al.*, 'Do they practice what we teach? A survey of manual handling practice amongst student nurses', *Journal of Clinical Nursing*, 12:2 (2003) 297–306.

Waters, T. *et al.*, 'NIOSH research efforts to prevent musculoskeletal disorders in the health care industry', *Orthopaedic Nursing* 25 (2006), 380–9.

II

Clinical Skills

At the end of this chapter the learner should be able to:

- **explain and define the vital signs**
- **discuss normal and abnormal values**
- **describe the appropriate equipment needed**
- **identify and explain the procedures used to obtain the vital signs**
- **describe how to record the vital signs accurately on a patient chart**
- **execute the measurement and accurate recording of vital signs**

Vital signs

Vital signs are taken by nurses and midwives in order to assess the most basic body functions. Vital signs may be called the observations or 'obs' (Iggulden *et al.*, 2009). It is essential that you are competent at executing each observation before you undertake it. An Bord Altranais (2008:1) stipulates that 'As a student, it is important that you do not undertake care for which you have not been prepared or for which you are not appropriately supervised.' Accuracy is also very important. Always report abnormal findings immediately. If unsure ask a colleague to recheck.

There are four vital signs which are standard in most medical settings:
- body temperature: **T**
- pulse rate (or heart rate): **P/ H.R.**
- blood pressure: **B.P.**
- respiratory rate: **R.R.**

In this chapter we will cover the observations listed above and also fluid balance.

Temperature

Body temperature represents the balance between heat gain and heat loss (Dougherty and Lister, 2008). The degree of heat of a body is measured by a thermometer.

Body temperature is usually around 36.8°C regardless of environmental changes. Slight variations occur (0.5° to 0.75°) in the morning and evening, when exercising, following eating and ovulation. Babies, young children and the elderly are particularly vulnerable to extremes of temperature.

The temperature-regulating centre is located in the hypothalamus and responds to the temperature of circulating blood and messages from thermoreceptors (Waugh and Grant, 2010).

Heat gain

Heat is produced in response to a drop in normal body temperature. Metabolic activity produces heat and other sources of heat include the skeletal muscles, the liver and the digestive organs.

When the skeletal muscles contract heat is produced (the more active the muscle the more heat produced). Shivering causes muscle contraction and therefore also leads to heat production.

The liver produces heat as it is very metabolically active, particularly after eating, peristalsis and chemical reactions in the digestive organs produce heat (Waugh and Grant, 2010).

Heat loss

The majority of heat loss occurs through the skin. Heat is lost by evaporation, radiation, conduction and convection.

- **Evaporation** of sweat cools the body.
- Heat **radiates** away from exposed parts of the body.
- **Conduction** occurs when clothes in direct contact with the skin absorb heat from the body.
- **Convection** occurs when exposed parts of the body heat air, which causes the air to rise and be replaced by cool air, setting up convection currents (Waugh and Grant, 2010).

Why do we record temperature?

- to obtain a baseline temperature for comparison with future recordings
- to monitor fluctuations in temperature – assessing health or illness

Monitoring temperature is an important aspect of the nursing/midwifery process. Accurate measurement is **very** important.

Patients that require temperature monitoring

- those with metabolic disorders
- post-operative patients
- critically ill patients
- those who are susceptible to infection
- those with infections
- in cases of blood transfusion

Types of thermometers

- Tympanic: an infra-red light source with a disposable cover is placed into the ear

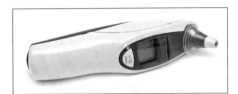

- Disposable: single-use strips that are usually placed on the skin (forehead)

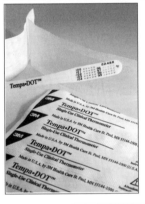

- Digital: check that the baseline reading is 34°C before use

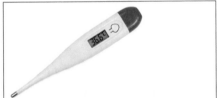

- Electronic: a sensor probe is attached to the skin (used in A&E, ITU)

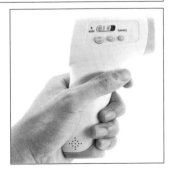

- Infra-red: a contactless infra-red light source is flashed on to the patient's forehead

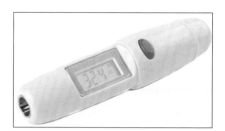

Recording sites
- Traditional sites
  - ‣ mouth
  - ‣ rectum
  - ‣ axillae
- New sites
  - ‣ ear
  - ‣ forehead

Considerations when selecting recording site
- Ear – tympanic thermometer
  - ‣ insert probe into ear canal
  - ‣ hygienic, non-invasive, quick recording
  - ‣ correct positioning is key
- Axillary
  - ‣ least desirable
  - ‣ difficult to get accurate readings – not close to major vessels
  - ‣ affected by environment
  - ‣ use same arm and place thermometer in the centre of axilla with arm firmly against side
- Oral
  - ‣ place thermometer in sublingual pocket at the base of the tongue
  - ‣ close to thermoreceptors
  - ‣ affected by food, fluids and smoking
- Rectal
  - ‣ often higher than oral
  - ‣ thought to be more accurate
  - ‣ invasive and time-consuming
  - ‣ rectal thermometer should be inserted at least 4 cm in adult to get accurate recording

Hyperthermia

A significant rise in body temperature is known as pyrexia or hyperthermia and is usually an indication of an infection. There are three grades of pyrexia:

- Low grade (normal to 38°C): indicates an inflammatory response due to mild infection, allergy or disturbance of body tissue such as surgery, injury or thrombosis.
- Moderate to high grade (38–40°C): can be caused by an infected wound or soft tissue injury.
- Hyperpyrexia (40°C and above): causes include bacteraemia, injury to the hypothalamus or high ambient temperature.

(Dougherty and Lister, 2008)

Treatment

Treatment will depend on the patient, their condition and prognosis, the probable cause and the grade of the hyperthermia. Treatments may include:

- Maintain close observation and seek medical advice.
- Monitor vital signs and fluid balance.
- Identify cause and treat, particularly if there is infection.
- Rehydrate with oral fluids (cold drinks but not ice) and/or mouthwashes.
- To improve patient's comfort, lower the room temperature; open a window if possible. Fans should not be used.
- Paracetamol – use with caution as it may slow down the automatic cooling functions of the body.

Hypothermia

Hypothermia is defined as a drop in body temperature below 35°C. Possible causes of hypothermia include:

- environmental exposure to cold weather
- medication such as Paracetamol, or alcohol, which can alter perception of cold, increase heat loss through vasodilation or block heat generation
- metabolic conditions such as hypoglycaemia, adrenal insufficiency
- surgery to the body surface or internal organs, exposure of which affects the vasoconstrictor response

Warning signs

- no complaints of feeling the cold even in a cold room
- drowsiness and apathy
- slurred speech and a husky voice
- skin that is cold to the touch, including the abdomen and under the arms
- a puffy face that may appear pale or gray in colour
- slow and shallow breathing

(Redfern and Ross, 2006)

Treatment

Treatment depends on the symptoms in each case. Medical assistance should always be sought.

- Mild hypothermia at home may be resolved by gently and passively rewarming at home.
  - ▸ Ensure there are no draughts and room temperature is between 25°C and 30°C.
  - ▸ Use light blankets; cover the head and neck to reduce further heat loss.
- When temperature is below 32°C:
  - ▸ active external rewarming can be given
  - ▸ use warm baths and heaters
- Always monitor carefully.

(Redfern and Ross, 2006)

Taking the temperature: procedure guidelines

Using a tympanic membrane thermometer

Procedure	Rationale
1. Explain and discuss the procedure with the patient.	To ensure the patient understands the procedure and can give informed consent.
2. Wash your hands.	Reduce risk of cross infection and contamination.
3. Document to ensure the same ear is used for future recordings.	Differences between the two ears can result in 1°C difference.
4. Remove unit from base unit, use a dry wipe if necessary.	Alcohol-based wipes can lead to a false low recording.

5. Place disposable probe cover on probe tip.	Cover protects tip of probe and is necessary for functioning of thermometer.
6. Gently place probe into ear canal, ensuring snug fit.	Prevent air from entering ear, giving a false low temperature.
7. Press and release scan button.	To commence instrument scanning.
8. Remove probe from ear when recording complete – usually indicated by bleeps.	Recording usually complete within two seconds.
9. Read the temperature display.	Document in chart.
10. Press eject button to discard probe cover and replace thermometer in unit.	Probe covers are single-use.

(Doughty and Lister, 2008:469–70)

ACTIVITY

In pairs using different types of thermometers, record your partner's temperature on two different devices. What do you observe?

Pulse

'The pulse is a wave of distension and elongation felt in an artery wall each time the left ventricle ejects blood into the circulatory system' (Waugh and Grant, 2010:90). The rate at which the heart beats can be counted by taking the pulse. The normal range is 60 to 80 beats per minute: the heart rate and the pulse should be the same.

The pulse can be felt most easily where an artery lies close to the surface of the body.

Pulse points

- temporal pulse
- radial pulse
- brachial pulse
- carotid pulse
- apical pulse
- femoral pulse
- popliteal pulse

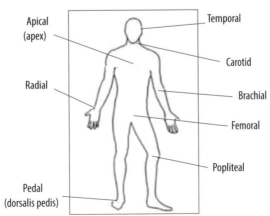

Apical (apex)

Radial

Pedal (dorsalis pedis)

Temporal

Carotid

Brachial

Femoral

Popliteal

- dorsalis pedis pulse
- posterior tibial pulse

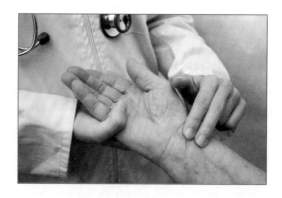

Common sites

- radial pulse in adults and older children
- apical pulse in babies and young children

Why take pulse rate?

- to assess heart rate, rhythm and strength of pulse
- to obtain baseline measurement as comparison against future recordings
- to monitor changes in pulse rate especially in patients who
    ‣ are pre/post-operation
    ‣ are receiving blood products
    ‣ have an infection
- to estimate the degree of fluid loss from the body

(Dougherty and Lister, 2008)

Three factors to assess when taking a pulse

Rate

The rate refers to the number of beats per minute. Normal rate is 60 to 80 beats per minute. Factors affecting pulse rate include:

- position – higher when standing than when lying down
- age – faster in infants and slows as we age
- gender – faster in women than men
- exercise – increases heart rate
- emotions – anxiety and excitement both increase the pulse rate in response to nervous system stimulation and release of adrenalin
- size of heart – a large heart may have a slower pulse rate compared with a smaller heart
- temperature – causes rises and falls in pulse rate

- disease – slowed by heart blockages, jaundice and increased pressure on the brain, increased by hyper-thyroidism, fever and haemorrhage

(Tucker, 2011; Waugh and Grant, 2010)

Rhythm

The rhythm refers to the sequence of beats, which is regular in a healthy individual. Defects in the conduction system of the heart cause irregularities. Fibrillation is a condition of irregular rapid contractions. Examples of different rhythms include:

- sinus rhythm – normal rhythm of heart
- sinus arrhythmia – irregularity of heart beat
- fibrillation – fast uncontrolled contraction of either upper (atrial) or lower (ventricular) chambers of the heart; can lead to cardiac arrest if left untreated

(Dougherty and Lister, 2008)

Any irregular heart rhythm must be reported.

Amplitude

Amplitude refers to the strength of the pulse and the elasticity of the arterial wall. The flexibility of the artery is affected by age; in an older person amplitude is affected by arteriosclerosis. A weak pulse may be an indication of bleeding, both internal and external, and assistance should be sought immediately.
(Dougherty and Lister, 2008)

Tachycardia

Tachycardia is defined as a heart rate greater than 100 bpm (beats per minute). It can occur in

- exercise, fever
- hypoxia
- congestive heart failure
- a fall in blood pressure
- pain, stress etc.

Bradycardia

Bradycardia is defined as an abnormally low heart rate, less than 60 bpm.

- indicates possible low body temperature, inadequate blood circulation to tissues

- occurs in
    - ▸ digitalis use – slows the heart
    - ▸ vomiting – stimulates the vagus nerve which reduces the rate
    - ▸ athletes – have well developed and efficient heart muscle

Taking the pulse: procedure guidelines

Action	Rationale
1. Explain and discuss the procedure with the patient.	To ensure the patient understands the procedure and can give informed consent.
2. Where possible measure the pulse under the same conditions each time. Ensure patient is comfortable.	To ensure continuity and consistency and to maintain comfort.
3. Place the first, second or third finger along the appropriate artery and press gently.	The fingertips are sensitive to touch. The thumb and forefinger have a pulse and may lead to incorrect recordings.
4. Press gently against the artery being used to record the pulse.	The radial artery is most commonly used as it is the most easily accessible.
5. The pulse should be counted for sixty seconds.	Sufficient time is required to detect irregularities.
6. Record the pulse rate.	Monitor differences, report irregularities to nursing/medical staff.

(Doughty and Lister, 2008, p. 446)

ACTIVITY

Find your radial pulse and count for a minute, then run on the spot for 30 seconds and repeat. How has exercise affected your pulse?

Respiration

Respiration refers to 'the exchange of gases between body cells and the environment' (Waugh and Grant, 2010:247). The respiratory system carries oxygen to the lungs where it enters the blood stream to travel throughout the body. Oxygen is necessary to create the energy for the metabolic processes that keep the body alive. Respiration involves two processes: breathing and gaseous exchange (Waugh and Grant, 2010). Effective control of respiration enables the body to maintain homeostasis over a wide range of physiological, environmental and pathological conditions.

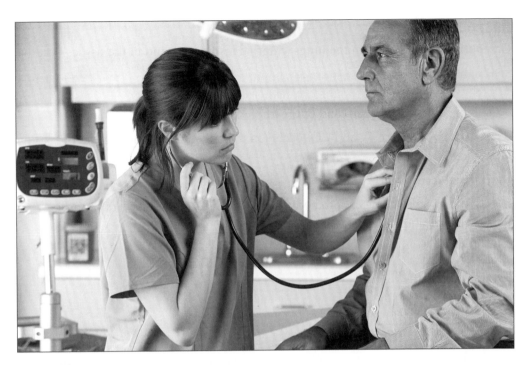

Breathing

Breathing is the regular inflation and deflation of the lungs which ensures the constant intake of oxygen and output of carbon dioxide.

Ventilation

Ventilation results from pressure changes transmitted from the thoracic cavity to the lungs, stimulating the cycle of respiration.

Cycle of respiration

The three parts of the cycle of respiration are inspiration, expiration and pause.

- **Inspiration** is initiated by contraction of the diaphragm and external intercostal muscles. The rib cage rises up and outwards expanding the lung's volume. Gases travel from an area of high pressure to low pressure – air rushes into the lungs. Inspiration takes about two seconds when the person is at rest.

- **Expiration** occurs as the inspiratory muscles relax and the lungs recoil. When the pressure inside the lungs is higher than outside the alveoli are compressed and expiration of gases occurs. Expiration takes about three seconds when the person is at rest.

- Before the cycle begins again there is a **pause**.

(Dougherty and Lister, 2008; Waugh and Grant, 2010)

Gaseous exchange

Gaseous exchange occurs in the lungs (external respiration) and in the tissues (internal respiration).

- external respiration

  ▸ breathing in (oxygen) and out (carbon dioxide)

  ▸ the exchange of O_2 and CO_2 occurs in the alveoli by the mechanism of diffusion

- internal respiration

  ▸ movement of oxygen into body tissues and cells and movement of carbon dioxide out of cells by the mechanism of diffusion

(Tucker, 2011)

Control of respiration

Respiratory centre

- located in the brain
- when motor neurons are stimulated the muscles contract and inspiration occurs
- when they are inhibited the muscles relax and expiration occurs
- generates basic rhythm but rate and depth are influenced by the body's needs

(Dougherty and Lister, 2008)

Chemical control

- chemoreceptors are located in the medulla oblongata (central) and in the aorta and carotid bodies (peripheral) and convey messages to the respiratory centre
- a rise in the amount of CO_2 in the blood supplying the respiratory centre stimulates the centre and breathing becomes faster and deeper
- in response to an increase in blood acidity, breathing rate increases, more CO_2 is expired, and blood pH returns to normal

(Waugh and Grant, 2010)

Other factors which influence breathing

- **Exercise** increases the body's demand for oxygen, therefore the rate and depth of breathing increase.
- **Temperature:** raised body temperature increases respiratory rate and low body temperature slows breathing.
- **Drugs and alcohol** reduce respiration rate.

- **Sleep** reduces respiration rate.
- **Emotion, pain and anxiety** cause an increase in respiratory rate.
- The *Hering-Breuer reflex* prevents over-inflation of the lungs.

(Waugh and Grant, 2010)

Why record respiration?

- to obtain a baseline respiratory rate for comparison
- to monitor changes in respiration and oxygenation
- to evaluate the patient's response to medications or treatments that affect the respiratory system

(Dougherty and Lister, 2008)

Three factors to assess when recording respiration

Rate

- ‣ normal rate: 14–18 respirations per minute (rpm)
- ‣ tachypneoa: increase in respiration rate – sign of rising temperature as the body tries to rid itself of excess heat
- ‣ bradypnoea: reduced respiration rate caused by depression of medulla by opiates or brain tumour

Depth

- ‣ volume of air moving in and out of lungs with each breath
- ‣ typical breathing is regular, automatic and requires no effort
- ‣ dyspnoea is undue breathlessness and discomfort with breathing

Pattern

- ‣ should be regular
- ‣ hyperventilation is excessive breathing caused by extreme exertion, fear, anxiety, diabetic ketoacidosis
- ‣ Cheyne-Stokes respiration is an abnormal pattern of breathing with a gradual increase in depth followed by decrease in respiration resulting in apnoea

(Dougherty and Lister, 2008)

Recording respiration: procedure guidelines

Observation	Rationale
1. Explain and discuss the procedure with the patient.	To ensure the patient understands the procedure and can give informed consent.
2. Where possible measure the pulse under the same conditions each time. Ensure the patient is comfortable.	To ensure continuity and consistency. To maintain comfort.
3. Assess rate and regularity of respiration.	Very slow or rapid breathing may be a sign of oxygenation or underlying change, for example due to sepsis.
4. Observe for signs of respiratory effort: • nasal flaring • pursed lips • use of neck and shoulder muscles.	These are signs that the patient is making an extra effort in breathing and indicate changes in respiratory status – report to nursing/medical staff.
5. Listen for cough or wheezing.	Dry cough – infection, congestive cardiac failure. Moist cough – chronic bronchitis. Wheezing – bronchospasm, obstruction.
6. Respirations should be counted for 60 seconds.	Sufficient time is required to detect irregularities.
7. Record the respiratory rate.	Monitor differences, report irregularities to nursing/medical staff.

(Dougherty and Lister, 2008:460)

ACTIVITY

In pairs: count your partner's pulse for one minute and then count their respirations for a further minute. Then tell your partner you are checking their respiration rate. What, if anything, do you notice?

✳ Blood pressure

'Blood pressure is force or pressure that the blood exerts on the wall of the blood vessels. Systemic arterial blood pressure maintains the essential flow of blood into and out of the organs' (Waugh and Grant, 2010:87). It is important to keep blood pressure within normal limits. The reading is recorded as a fraction: Systolic/Diastolic.

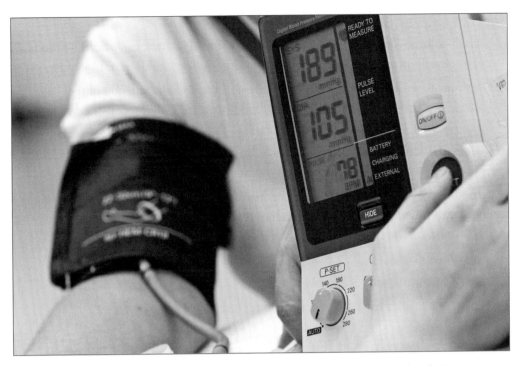

A reading of 120/80 mmHg is considered normal blood pressure (Irish Heart Foundation, 2012). However blood pressure can fluctuate and still be considered normal.

Systolic pressure

This is the peak pressure of the blood in the arteries and is caused by the contraction of the ventricle. It averages around 120 mmHg in adults.

Diastolic pressure

When the heart is resting following the ejection of blood the pressure is much lower in the arteries, usually about 80 mmHg in adults.
(Waugh and Grant, 2010)

Why do we check blood pressure?

- to obtain a baseline for comparison against future readings
- to monitor fluctuations in blood pressure

Factors that affect blood pressure

- Blood volume – normally at a consistent level but if haemhorrage occurs blood volume will drop affecting cardiac output and leading to a drop in blood pressure.
- Peripheral resistance – determined by the constriction and dilation of the arterioles; vasodilation causes a fall in blood pressure and vasoconstriction causes it to rise.
- Vessel elasticity – fibrous tissue replaces elastic tissue as we age making it harder for blood to pass through the vessels, increasing blood pressure.
- Condition of the heart muscle – if the heart muscle is less efficient it has to work harder to function, causing a rise in blood pressure.

Age-related factors

- Systolic pressure increases as we age.
- There is a smaller increase in diastolic pressure as we age.

Environmental factors

- Stress increases blood pressure.
- A diet high in salt, processed foods and animal fats leads to an increase in blood pressure.
- Medication can help regulate blood pressure in chronic hypertensive patients.
- Disease will affect the functioning of the heart.

Hypotension

Hypotension is defined in adults as a systolic blood pressure below 100 mmHg, though this can be a 'normal reading' for an individual.

- Controlled or induced: blood pressure may be artificially lowered for surgery, to reduce blood flow to the operation site.
- Postural: there may be a temporary lowering of blood pressure when a person stands up, resulting in a feeling of giddiness or fainting.

Hypertension

Hypertension is defined as a blood pressure reading greater than 140/90 mmHg.

- Diagnosis of hypertension is made when an average of two or more readings is recorded at rest several days apart followed by 24-hour blood pressure monitoring, usually at home.

- If the readings exceed the upper levels considered normal for that person they are considered hypertensive.

(IHF, 2012)

White-coat hypertension

Around 25 per cent of patients having their blood pressure checked in hospital or at a doctor's surgery exhibit 'white-coat syndrome', when their anxiety about having their blood pressure checked causes a rise in the reading.
(IHF, 2012)

Advice for hypertensive patient

- stop smoking
- reduce salt intake and eat less processed food
- lose weight and maintain a healthy weight
- become more active
- cut down on alcohol
- increase intake of fruit and vegetables

(IHF, 2012)

Recording equipment
Manual sphygmomanometers – Aneroid

- A mechanical device that measures the cuff pressure using a bellows connected to the cuff via rubber tubing.
- The pressure inside the bellows is transferred to a dial via a system of levers and gears.
- Common errors when using this device:
  ‣ systematic error – lack of concentration, poor hearing
  ‣ failure to interpret the korotkoff sounds correctly
  ‣ tendency to record blood pressures ending in '0' or '5'
  ‣ bias – recording a reading you were expecting for the patient
- Cuff
  ‣ encircles the arm and encloses an inflatable rubber bladder
  ‣ secured around the arm usually by velcro

- Control valve
  - allows the passage of air; when closed it should maintain air at a constant level and when released it should allow a steady fall in the level of air
- Stethoscope
  - ear piece and diaphragm
  - it is possible to identify the five phases of blood pressure
  - the diaphragm should be placed over the point of maximum pulsation

(Dougherty and Lister, 2008)

Korotkoff sounds

When executing a blood pressure recording you are listening for the Korotkoff Sounds. There are five phases:

1. The appearance of faint, clear tapping sounds which gradually increase in intensity.
2. The softening of sounds, which may become swishing.
3. The return of sharper sounds which become crisper but never fully regain the intensity of phase 1 sounds.
4. The distinct muffling sound which becomes soft and blowing.
5. The point at which all sound ceases.

The first sound is the systolic reading and the last sound is the diastolic.

Taking blood pressure: procedure guidelines

Action		Rationale
1.	Explain to the patient that blood pressure is to be taken and discuss the procedure.	To ensure the patient understands the procedure and can give informed consent.
2.	Allow patient to rest for 3 minutes if lying or seated, 1 minute if standing.	To ensure accurate reading, usually taken sitting.
3.	Ensure that the upper arm is supported and positioned at heart level, with palm facing upward.	To ensure accurate reading.
4.	Ensure tight or restrictive clothing is removed from the arm.	To obtain correct reading.
5.	Use a cuff that covers 80% of the circumference of the arm.	To obtain correct reading.

6.	Apply the cuff snugly around the arm, ensuring the centre of the bladder covers the brachial artery.	To obtain correct reading.
7.	Position the manometer within 1 m of the patient and where it can be seen at eye level.	To prevent tubing hanging down and being caught by another object.
8.	Instruct the patient to stop eating or talking during procedure.	Eating or talking can cause an inaccurate blood pressure reading.
9.	Inflate the cuff until the radial pulse can no longer be felt, this provides an estimate of systolic pressure. Deflate the cuff and wait 15–30 seconds before continuing.	A low systolic pressure may be reported in patients who have an auscultatory gap. This is when Korotkoff sounds disappear shortly after the systolic pressure is heard and resume well above what corresponds to diastolic pressure.
10.	Inflate the cuff to a pressure 30 mmHg higher than the estimated systolic pressure.	Pressure exerted by the inflated cuff prevents the blood from flowing through the artery.
11.	The diaphragm of the stethoscope should be placed over the pulse point in the brachial artery.	Apply just enough pressure to keep it in place; too much pressure can distort the sounds.
12.	Do not tuck the diaphragm under the cuff.	To prevent inaccurate recording.
13.	Deflate the cuff at 2 mmHg per second or per heart beat.	Too slow deflation causes congestion pain and false reading.
14.	The measurement of systolic BP is when a minimum of two clear repetitive sounds can be heard. Diastolic pressure is recorded at the point when the sound can no longer be heard.	To ensure that an accurate reading is obtained.
15.	Record reading noting arm used and report findings to medical staff.	To ensure consistency and that appropriate action is taken.
16.	Remove equipment and clean after use.	To reduce risk of cross infection.

(Dougherty and Lister, 2008:454–5)

ACTIVITY

Practise taking blood pressures in pairs, ensuring you communicate effectively with your 'patient'. This skill will take time and a lot of practice.

Fluid balance

'Fluid balance is maintaining the correct amount of fluid in the body. It is the continuance of the fluid input and output of the body. Fluid balance can alter with disease and illness' (Mooney, 2007).

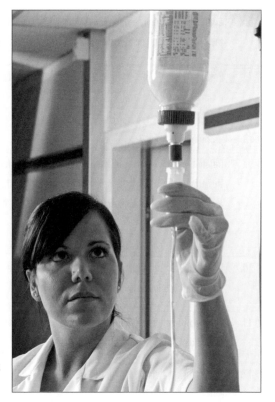

As long as the mechanisms for stimulating thirst in the brain (osmoreceptors) and kidney function remain intact, the body is able to maintain total fluid volume.

Water as a percentage of total body weight changes from foetal (80 per cent) to adulthood (approximately 65 per cent). A reduction in body fluids can have major effects on the body: a reduction of 5 per cent will cause thirst, a reduction of 8 per cent will cause illness and a 10 per cent reduction in fluid can cause death (Carroll, 2000).

Why do we record fluid balance?

- to assess intake of fluids
  - orally
  - intravenously
  - naso-gastrically
  - parenterally
- to assess output
- to maintain homeostasis (balance)

Potential gains

- oral intake:
  - fluids
  - nutritional supplements
  - bowel preparations

- IV intake:
  - ▸ colloids and crystalloids
  - ▸ feeds
  - ▸ drugs

Expected losses

- measurable
  - ▸ urine (measure hourly if necessary)
  - ▸ GI (stool, stoma, drains, tubes)
- insensible
  - ▸ sweat
  - ▸ exhaled

Disturbance in fluid balance

- fluid depletion or loss is called hypovolaemia
- fluid gain or overload is called hypervolaemia

Factors that cause fluid loss or gain

Fluid loss/depletion

- diarrhoea
- vomiting
- sweating/fever
- haemorrhage
- diuretics
- excessive urination

Fluid gain/overload

- congestive cardiac failure
- renal failure
- high sodium intake
- cirrhosis of the liver
- over infusion of intravenous fluids

All of the above can be symptoms of disease and illness (Mooney, 2007).

Observations related to fluid balance

Observation	Fluid depletion	Fluid overload
Weight	Loss	Gain
Blood pressure	Lowered smaller pulse pressure	Normal or raised
Respirations	Rapid, shallow	Rapid, moist cough
Pulse	Rapid, weak, thready	Rapid
Urine output	Reduced, concentrated	Increased or decreased if heart is failing
Skin	Dry, less elastic	Oedematous
Saliva	Thick, viscous	Copious, frothy
Tongue	Dry, coated	Moist
Thirst	Present	No disturbance
Face	Sunken eyes (severe depletion)	Peri-orbital oedema
Temperature	May be raised	No disturbance

(Place and Field, 1997)

Recording fluid balance: procedure guidelines

Action	Rationale
1. Explain to the patient that you are recording their fluid intake and output and discuss the procedure.	To ensure the patient understands the procedure and can give informed consent.
2. Include the patient's history, clinical observation and laboratory results if relevant.	To ensure holistic accurate measurement is obtained.
3. Record the input and output in the fluid balance chart.	To ensure accuracy.
4. Report findings.	To maintain safety.

ACTIVITY

Jack is 89 years old. His daily fluid input and output are recorded below.

Cup/glass = 150 ml, mug = 200 ml

Complete the following fluid balance table:

Input	Output	
Morning: 1 cup of tea	7am:	300mls
1 glass of orange juice	11am:	200mls
½ glass of water with his medication		
Lunch: 1 glass of milk	1pm:	150mls
½ cup of tea		
Afternoon: 1 cup of tea	3pm:	200mls
Teatime: 1 cup of tea	5pm:	150mls
Supper: 1 mug of hot milk	9pm:	150mls
Total: _____	**Total:** _____	

What does the above finding tell you?

Recording observations on patients' charts

Observation charts may vary between different healthcare facilities but they are generally of similar layout and contain basic information.

The chart must contain **patient details** clearly printed or using a printed label:

- patient's name
- address
- hospital number
- date of birth

Before you start the recording of vital signs you must ensure you have the correct patient by asking the patient, checking their hospital identity band and ensuring you have the corresponding chart.

Date and time

- The date should be recorded in full: day, month and year.
- The time should be recorded using the twenty-four-hour clock: record the exact time of the observation.

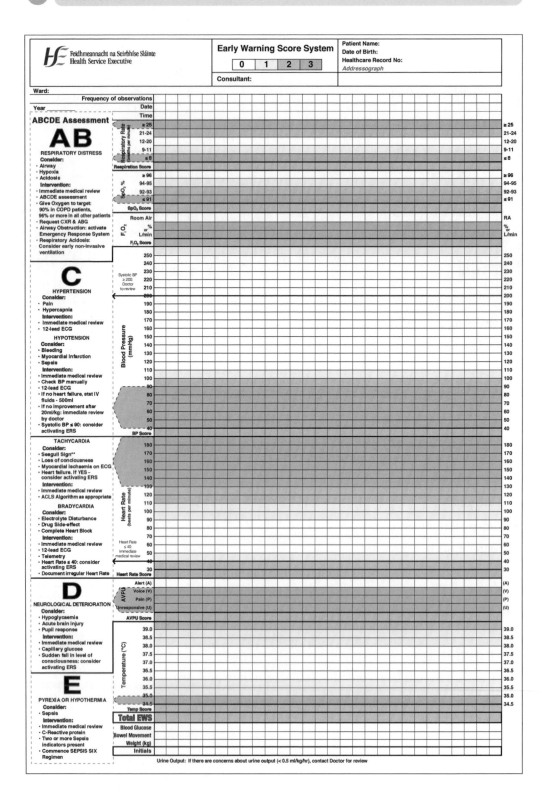

Temperature

Place a dot on the chart corresponding with the temperature measurement, e.g. 36.5°C, and join up to the previous recording with a single line (Iggulden *et al.*, 2009).

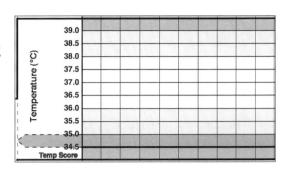

Pulse

You must count the pulse rate for 60 seconds to obtain an accurate result. Place a dot on the chart corresponding with the pulse measurement and join up to the previous recording with a single line (Iggulden *et al.*, 2009).

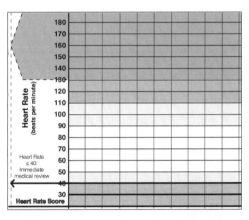

Respirations

Similarly respiration rate is counted for 60 seconds and may be recorded with a dot joined to the previous recording with a single line, or as a figure, e.g. 16 rpm.

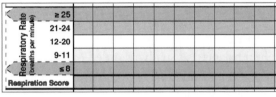

Blood pressure

Methods of recording blood pressure reading vary. It is important to identify the systolic and diastolic readings and join them either by a dotted line or by a straight line (Iggulden *et al.*, 2009).

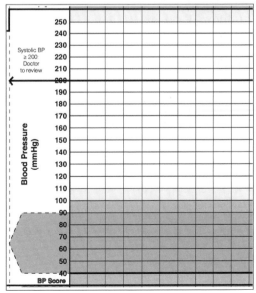

Recording fluid balance

The fluid balance chart must contain patient details clearly printed or using a printed label:

- patient's name
- address
- hospital number
- date of birth

Fluid balance is usually recorded over a twenty-four-hour period, for example starting at 08.00 hrs and finishing 07.59 hrs the following morning.

Fluid intake comprises intravenous fluids, oral fluids and nasogastric feeds if applicable.
Output involves urine, vomit, drains, nasogastric if applicable.

Both columns are totalled and the output is subtracted from the input to assess whether the patient is sufficiently hydrated or dehydrated.

Fluid Balance Chart
Date: _____

Name _____

Hosp No _____

Instructions:

Time	Intake (record in mL)					Output (record in mL)				
	Oral	PEG NG	Blood Products IV Meds	IV Fluids SC Fluids	Totals *Cumulative*	Urine	Aspiration Vomit	Colostomy Drains	Totals *Cumulative*	
08.00										
09.00										
10.00										
11.00										
12.00										
13.00										
14.00										
15.00										
16.00										
17.00										
18.00										
19.00										
Day Totals =										
20.00										
21.00										
22.00										
23.00										
24.00										
01.00										
02.00										
03.00										
04.00										
05.00										
06.00										
07.00										
24 Hr Totals										

Total Intake (mL)		Balance (mL) 24 hours	Positive:
Total Output (mL)			Negative:

Revision
Temperature
1. What is normal body temperature?
2. List four sites that can be used to monitor body temperature.
3. Define the following terms:
    *   hypothermia
    *   pyrexia
4. List the causes of hypothermia and pyrexia.

Pulse
5. What is the average resting pulse rate of an adult?
6. List three characteristics you would note when checking a pulse rate.
7. What could an increase in pulse rate indicate?
8. What could a slow pulse rate indicate?

Respiration
9. What is the average respiratory rate of an adult?
10. What information would you require about a client before taking their respiratory rate?
11. List three characteristics you would note when checking respiratory rate.

Blood pressure
12. Why do we check blood pressure?
13. Identify the two pieces of equipment needed to check blood pressure and their purpose.
14. What is the medical term for high blood pressure?
15. What is the medical term for low blood pressure?
16. Identify signs or symptoms of low blood pressure and high blood pressure.

Fluid balance
17. What does the term fluid balance refer to?
18. Why is it important to monitor and record fluid balance?

References

An Bord Altranais, *Guidance for Nursing Students*, Dublin: ABA 2008, 1.

Carroll, H., 'Fluid and electrolytes' in Sheppard, M. and Wright, M., eds, *Principles and Practice of High Dependency Nursing*, Edinburgh: Baillière Tindall 2000.

Dougherty, L. and Lister, S., *The Royal Marsden Hospital Manual of Clinical Nursing Procedures,* 7th ed., Oxford: Blackwell Publishing 2008, 446, 454–5, 460, 469–70.

Iggulden, H. *et al.*, *Clinical Skills – The Essence of Caring*, London: McGraw Hill 2009.

Irish Heart Foundation, *Manage your Blood Pressure*, Dublin: IHF 2012.

Jevon, P., 'How to ensure patient observations lead to effective management of patients with pyrexia', *Nursing Times*, 106:1 (2010), available at www.nursingtimes.net (accessed 21/7/13).

Mooney, G., 'Fluid balance' available at www.nursingtimes.net/nursing-practice/clinical-zones/cardiology/fluid-balance/199391.article (2007) (accessed 22/7/13).

Place, B. and Field, D., 'The management of fluid balance', *Nursing Times*, 93:44 (1997), 46–8.

Redfern, S. and Ross, F., *Nursing Older People*, 5th ed., Edinburgh: Churchill Livingstone 2006.

Tucker, L., *An Introductory Guide to Anatomy and Physiology*, London: EMS Publishing 2011, Chapters 2, 5, 11.

Waugh, A. and Grant, A., *Ross and Wilson Anatomy and Physiology in Health and Illness*, 11th ed., Edinburgh: Churchill Livingstone 2010, 87, 90, 247.

Index

Page numbers in **bold italic** indicate charts, diagrams, etc.